The Universe of Hearing - System, Technologies, Interdisciplinarity, and Challenges

Edited by Milaine Dominici Sanfins and Piotr Henryk Skarzynski

Published in London, United Kingdom

The Universe of Hearing - System, Technologies, Interdisciplinarity, and Challenges
http://dx.doi.org/10.5772/intechopen.1009704
Edited by Milaine Dominici Sanfins and Piotr Henryk Skarzynski

Contributors
Adam Pabiś, Cilmara Cristina Alves da Costa Levy, Dalian Ding, Daniela Gil, Fernanda Soares Aurélio Patatt, Karina Carlesso Pagliarin, Liling Li, Lisiane Holdefer, Milaine Dominici Sanfins, Oluwasola Timothy, Oyinwola Oluwafisayo, Ozioko Obialunamma, Peng Li, Piotr Henryk Skarzynski, Rochele Martins Machado, Thiago Silva Almeida de Souza

First published in London, United Kingdom, 2026 by IntechOpen
IntechOpen is the global imprint of INTECHOPEN LIMITED, registered in England and Wales, registration number: 11086078, 167-169 Great Portland Street, London, W1W 5PF, United Kingdom

For EU product safety concerns: IN TECH d.o.o., Prolaz Marije Krucifikse Kozulić 3, 51000 Rijeka, Croatia, info@intechopen.com or visit our website at intechopen.com.

British Library Cataloguing-in-Publication Data
A catalogue record for this book is available from the British Library

The Universe of Hearing - System, Technologies, Interdisciplinarity, and Challenges
Edited by Milaine Dominici Sanfins and Piotr Henryk Skarzynski
p. cm.
Print ISBN 978-1-80631-130-9
Online ISBN 978-1-80631-129-3
eBook (PDF) ISBN 978-1-80631-131-6

Meet the editors

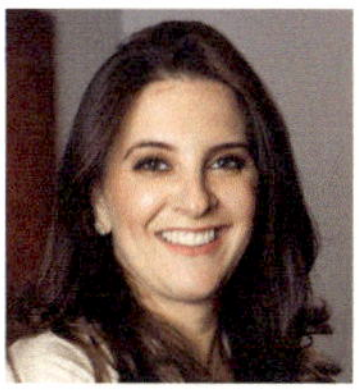

Milaine Dominici Sanfins is an Associate Professor in the Department of Speech-Language Pathology at the Federal University of São Paulo (UNIFESP), Brazil, with a specialization in audiology, electroacoustics, and electrophysiology. She obtained her Ph.D. in Child and Adolescent Health from UNICAMP and the Università degli Studi di Ferrara (2017), followed by a postdoctoral fellowship at the World Hearing Center in Poland (2021). She currently serves on the Research Ethics Committee and the Teaching and Research Commission of the Brazilian Academy of Audiology (2024-2026). Her research encompasses neuroaudiology, neonatal screening, pediatric and adolescent diagnosis, otoacoustic emissions, electrophysiology, and auditory interventions, supported by over 65 peer-reviewed articles and 16 book chapters. Sanfins has achieved recognition by promoting international collaborations and serving in editorial roles in audiology and neuroscience.

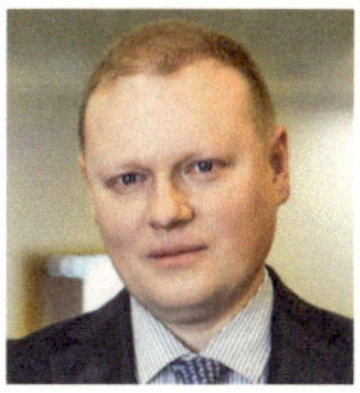

Prof. Piotr H. Skarzynski, MD, Ph.D., MSc, is a specialist in ENT, paediatric ENT, audiology, phoniatrics, and public health. He conducts research at the World Hearing Center of the Institute of Physiology and Pathology of Hearing. He participated in the WHO's World Hearing Forum announcement and has served as Board Member of the International Society for Telemedicine and e-Health, President of the International Advisory Board of the American Academy of Otolaryngology-Head and Neck Surgery, and Vice-President of the Hearing Group. He is an Honorary Member of the ORL Danube Society and Société Française d'Oto-Rhino-Laryngologie, and a Member of the Council of Poland's National Science Centre. His research interests include ENT surgery, otology, hearing devices, telemedicine, robotics, and hearing screening across multiple continents.

Contents

Preface

Auditory perception is a fundamental sense crucial for human development, essential for verbal communication, social interaction, learning, and overall quality of life throughout all stages of existence. In recent decades, advances in audiological science and technology have greatly enhanced our understanding of hearing mechanisms, the aetiology of hearing loss, and therapeutic approaches for its prevention, diagnosis, and rehabilitation.

This compilation draws on insights from experts across various nations, offering a thorough and contemporary perspective on key topics in clinical audiology. This work's chapters illustrate the complexity and multidisciplinary approach required to address the diverse conditions that impact the auditory system from childhood to adulthood across challenging clinical contexts.

The work commences with a chapter on the implementation of universal neonatal hearing screening in remote regions, focusing on a pilot study conducted in Nigeria and underscoring the challenges faced by developing nations. Notwithstanding the obstacles posed by infrastructure, awareness, and follow-up systems, the study illustrates the viability of this crucial practice, underscoring the need for investments in public health and targeted interventions.

An extensive examination of the correlation between hearing loss and infectious diseases is undertaken, emphasising how both congenital and acquired pathogens, such as cytomegalovirus, rubella, bacterial meningitis, and more recently, COVID-19, can irreparably impair auditory function, particularly in children. Chapter 2 underscores the imperative of enhancing vaccination initiatives, instituting universal and ongoing neonatal hearing assessments, monitoring for drug-induced ototoxicity, and bolstering educational campaigns, especially in low- and middle-income nations where these infections are major preventable causes of deafness and irreversible hearing loss.

Chapter 3 focuses on antioxidation, and the inner ear provides a crucial perspective on the application of antioxidants in the prevention and management of sensorineural hearing loss. The authors caution against the "antioxidant paradox," showing that indiscriminate or excessive interventions can paradoxically exacerbate cellular damage. This discourse is crucial for directing more accurate and safer therapeutic approaches, predicated on the targeted modulation of oxidative stress. The chapter establishes a robust scientific foundation for realigning future therapeutic strategies, shifting from generic free-radical elimination to targeted and personalised interventions.

The collection also examines the significant relationship between hearing loss and cognitive decline in Chapter 4, a subject of growing importance given global population ageing. Hearing difficulties can exacerbate cognitive overload, thereby accelerating neurodegenerative processes that impact memory, attention, language, and executive functions. The authors underscore the critical necessity of employing cognitive assessment instruments specifically tailored for individuals with hearing loss, which mitigate auditory biases through visual and written stimuli. This text discusses scientific evidence indicating that hearing rehabilitation with hearing aids can maintain or enhance cognitive performance, while also highlighting critical deficiencies, particularly the lack of suitable tools for individuals with low educational attainment. It concludes that interdisciplinary strategies combining hearing rehabilitation, cognitive stimulation, and ongoing monitoring are vital for reducing risks and fostering cognitive health during ageing.

Hearing rehabilitation in complex cases is conducted with careful consideration of the clinical specifics associated with conditions such as auditory neuropathy, Down syndrome, non-progressive chronic encephalopathies, and autism spectrum disorder.

Chapter 5 introduces neuromodulation as a novel and crucial therapeutic option for tinnitus management, particularly in cases unresponsive to standard treatments. The authors examine primary neuromodulation techniques, providing evidence from randomised clinical trials that alleviate tinnitus-related suffering and demonstrating a favourable safety profile and a low incidence of adverse effects. The chapter underscores that, notwithstanding significant progress, there is an imperative requirement for comprehensive research to standardise protocols, delineate responder profiles, formulate effective combinations, and amalgamate neuromodulation with audiological and psychobehavioral approaches.

Chapter 6 encompasses ARC (Adaptive Synaptic Adaptation) Therapy, a novel tinnitus treatment predicated on the notion that tinnitus serves as an auditory counterpart to phantom pain. This condition arises when abrupt hearing loss hinders prompt neural reorganisation, resulting in the structural integrity of the neuronal population in the spiral ganglion and cochlear nuclei while maintaining functional hyperactivity, thereby producing the sensation of phantom sound. The clinical study results indicated a decrease in tinnitus severity and emphasised the significance of optimising patients' metabolic health in patient care. The author asserts that ARC constitutes a promising, safe, and non-invasive therapeutic approach, with intentions for global expansion through a mobile application for automated diagnosis and programming, as well as integration with contemporary hearing aids that facilitate amplification beyond 8 kHz.

The last chapter underscores the necessity for therapeutic individualisation, asserting that the standardisation of protocols is no longer permissible given recent diagnostic advancements. The author underscores the essential significance of interdisciplinary collaboration among audiologists, speech therapists, occupational therapists, educators, and families to formulate individualised therapeutic plans that address each child's unique needs, taking into account cultural, educational, and developmental factors, thereby fostering not only auditory enhancement but also linguistic, cognitive, psychosocial development, and the successful social integration of these children.

Milaine Dominici Sanfins
Professor of Department of Speech-Hearing-Language,
Universidade Federal de São Paulo,
São Paulo, Brazil

Piotr Henryk Skarzynski
Department of Otolaryngology,
Centrum Słuchu i Mowy Medincus,
Warsaw, Poland

Section 1

Prevention and Early Diagnosis

Chapter 1

Challenges of a Universal Newborn Hearing Screening in Remote Settings: A Pilot Study

Oyinwola Oluwafisayo, Ozioko Obialunamma and Oluwasola Timothy

Abstract

Universal newborn hearing screening (UNHS) is a global public health initiative designed to facilitate early identification of infants with permanent congenital or early-onset hearing loss, enabling timely intervention and rehabilitation. However, numerous challenges hinder the establishment of sustainable programs in developing countries. This study explored the feasibility of implementing UNHS and identified barriers to its adoption in a rural Nigerian hospital. All infants delivered within or outside the facility were eligible for hearing screening. The Otoport Advance OAE + ABR screener (Otodynamics®, UK) was used to assess both ears in a two-stage protocol comprising distortion product otoacoustic emissions, followed immediately by automated auditory brainstem response. Outcome variables included screening coverage, first-screen refer rate, rescreening rate, referral rate at rescreen, and dropout rate. Of 163 mothers or caregivers who provided informed consent, 152 newborns were sampled, and after data cleaning, 132 were analysed. Coverage was 17.2%. The first-screen refer rate for both tests was 28.8% (n = 38) in one or both ears, the rescreen refer rate was 3.03% (n = 4), and the dropout rate was 73.7% (n = 28). These findings were attributed to low awareness and acceptance, inadequate screening units and staff, weak data management and tracking systems, and poor screening infrastructure. In conclusion, although screening coverage was low and the dropout rate high, the referral rate (3.03%) was within the acceptable threshold (<4%). This study demonstrates that UNHS is feasible in remote settings, and existing challenges are surmountable through targeted interventions and improved health-system support.

Keywords: hearing screening, newborn, UNHS, rural, hospital, low-resource settings, AABR, DPOAE, pilot study

1. Introduction

Universal newborn hearing screening (UNHS) is now a critical component of early hearing detection and intervention (EHDI) programs in high-income countries, aimed at the prompt detection of permanent congenital or early-onset hearing loss

(PCEHL) for timely intervention and rehabilitation. Despite the proven benefits of early identification, most developing nations have yet to implement nationwide UNHS programs due to systemic barriers such as insufficient infrastructure, weak policy frameworks, absence of supportive legislation, shortage of trained personnel, and inadequate funding for health services [1]. About two decades ago, Olusanya et al. reported challenges to the success of UNHS programs in developing countries, including limited funding, manpower shortages, inadequate support services, low public awareness, and uncertainty regarding the commitment from healthcare practitioners [2]. In the post-COVID-19 era, global economic instability and inflation have exacerbated these pre-existing challenges, diverting limited resources away from preventive programs such as hearing screening towards more immediate public health concerns [3]. However, the prevalence of hearing loss remains high in the country [4, 5] with dire consequences if unaddressed and the severity of impact being influenced by age of onset, degree of hearing loss, age of identification and intervention, and the environment, which includes access to services such as hearing technology, special education, and sign language [6].

2. Main chapter body text

2.1 Background

The ability to hear is often taken for granted, yet hearing loss remains the most common form of sensory impairment worldwide and is frequently referred to as a 'hidden disability' because it is neither visible nor immediately recognised. Hearing, or auditory perception, refers to the ability to detect and interpret sound vibrations through the auditory system [7]. Hearing loss refers to a reduced ability to perceive sound compared with an individual with normal hearing, which has been demonstrated to begin in the early second trimester, with foetal responses first elicited at lower frequencies and subsequently at higher frequencies (up to 1,000 Hz) [8, 9]. As gestation advances, responses occur at progressively lower sound intensities, indicating increasing auditory sensitivity associated with the maturation of the cochlear and neural pathways. Consequently, by birth, the auditory system is functionally mature, providing the physiological basis for UNHS.

Permanent congenital or early-onset hearing impairment occurs at birth or within the first 28 days of life and typically represents pre-lingual hearing impairment [2]. Permanent congenital or early-onset hearing loss significantly contributes to speech delay, impaired language development, and reduced educational attainment in children, particularly in low- and middle-income countries (LMICs) [1, 8]. Approximately 40% of childhood hearing loss has a genetic origin, whereas the remaining cases result from preventable causes such as infections, birth asphyxia, ototoxic medications, and neonatal jaundice – conditions that are more prevalent in developing countries [8], such as Nigeria, where government health expenditure is low, as shown in **Figure 1** [10].

2.2 Epidemiology

Globally, over 360 million people are estimated to live with disabling hearing loss, of whom approximately 32 million (9%) are children. World Health Organisation

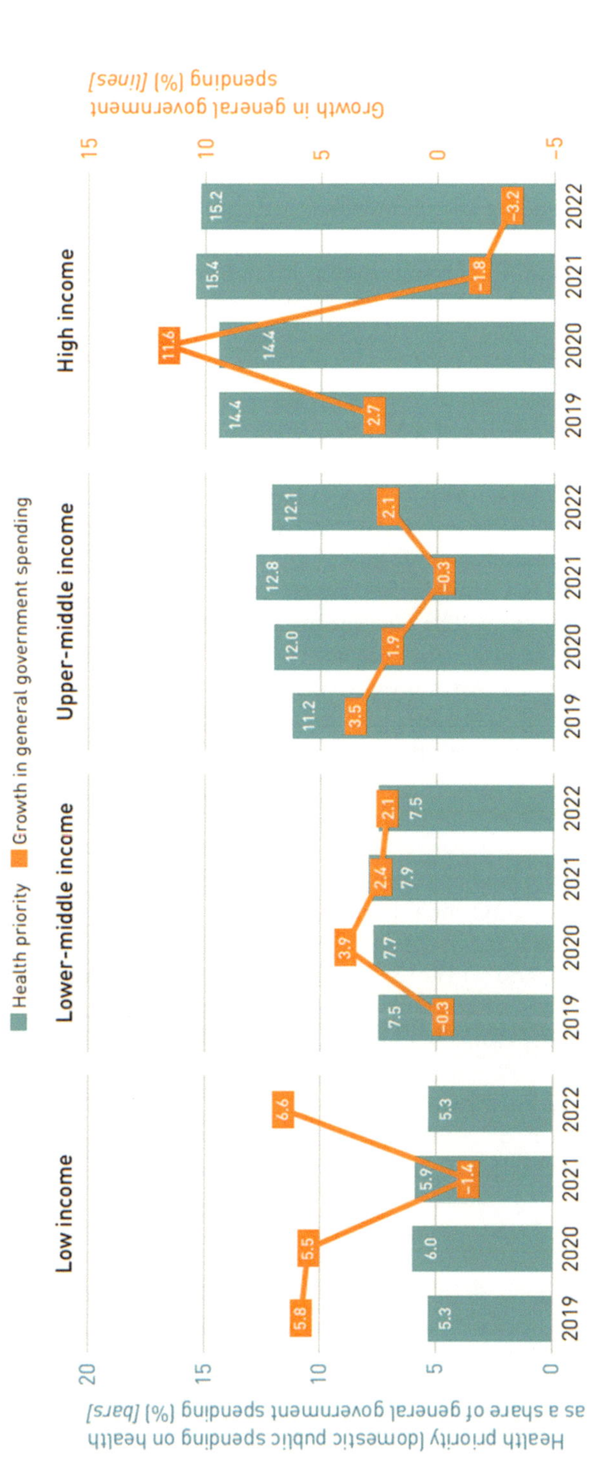

Figure 1.
Health priority and growth in general government spending by income group, 2019–2022. (source: World Health Organization, Global Health Expenditure Database, 2024).

(WHO) projections indicate that by 2050, one in 10 people will experience disabling hearing loss, with a disproportionate burden borne by populations in sub-Saharan Africa and other LMICs [6, 8]. In Nigeria, studies conducted over the past two decades report a high prevalence of hearing loss, with an estimated incidence of 28 per 1000 live births in a community-based study [11] and 5.5 per 1000 in a hospital-based study [12] conducted in Lagos. Despite these findings, a nationwide UNHS program has not been implemented. The WHO recommends that countries with diverse health systems adopt newborn and infant hearing screening tailored to their economic and social realities [1]. However, in those countries where the UNHS has not been established, the common obstacles identified include a lack of locally adapted guidelines, financial constraints, and insufficient political commitment [1].

2.3 Rationale

Although Nigeria introduced a National Policy and Strategic Plan for Ear and Hearing Care in 2018, specifying strategies for early detection and intervention, the implementation of universal hearing screening remains largely theoretical [13]. Previous efforts within the country [14–17] have been limited to targeted screenings for high-risk infants based on the Joint Committee on Infant Hearing (JCIH) guidelines [18], which fail to identify a substantial proportion of affected newborns without obvious risk factors. The current pilot study was therefore designed to explore the feasibility of implementing a structured UNHS program in a resource-limited, remote healthcare setting. By identifying context-specific challenges and testing practical, scalable solutions, this study aims to provide an evidence base for national-level program adaptation and integration into routine neonatal care.

2.4 Definitions

Normal hearing is defined as a threshold of 20 decibels (dB) or better in both ears, while the WHO defines functional hearing impairment in children as an unaided permanent hearing loss greater than 30 dB in the better ear, averaged over frequencies of 0.5, 1, 2, and 4 kHz [6, 19]. Disabling hearing loss refers to hearing loss greater than 40 dB in the better hearing ear in adults and a hearing loss greater than 30 dB in the better hearing ear in children [20]. Although the WHO defines functional hearing impairment in children as a permanent unaided hearing loss exceeding 30 dB in the better ear [6], this definition excludes children with milder losses between 21 and 29 dB, who may still experience communication, social, and developmental challenges [1].

2.5 The burden of PCEHL

Globally, approximately 5.3% (360 million people) of the population lives with disabling hearing loss, of which sub-Saharan Africa accounts for roughly 9% (32.4 million) [20]. Children aged 0–14 years represent nearly 1.9% of this group (≈600,000 children) [20]. The prevalence of congenital or early-onset sensorineural hearing loss ranges from 0.5 to 5 per 1000 newborns worldwide but is notably higher in LMICs [1]. Sub-Saharan Africa ranks third globally in the prevalence of disabling childhood hearing loss, with rates nearly twice those observed in high-income regions [20]. In Nigeria, the national prevalence of disabling hearing loss has been estimated at

6.7%, yet the under-five prevalence remains largely undocumented due to the absence of a structured newborn hearing screening program (NHSP) capable of generating population-level data [13]. Most existing evidence derives from studies among school-aged children, retrospectively extrapolated to the neonatal period. Earlier research reported a PCEHL prevalence of 6 per 1000 live births (0.6%), while more recent hospital-based studies employing one- or two-stage screening have observed bilateral hearing loss rates between 6.5% and 8% [4, 5, 15].

2.6 The goals of UNHSP

The American Academy of Pediatrics, in line with the JCIH, endorses the universal detection of infant hearing loss as a public-health imperative. The principal objective of a universal newborn hearing screening program (UNHSP) is to ensure that all newborns are screened using physiologic methods capable of identifying significant bilateral hearing loss – defined as thresholds of 35 dB or worse in the better ear [21]. The definition encompasses bilateral or unilateral permanent conductive, sensory, and neural (auditory neuropathy/dyssynchrony) hearing impairments in infants admitted to the neonatal intensive care unit [18]. The EHDI framework seeks to maximise linguistic competence and literacy outcomes among children who are deaf or hard of hearing [18]. To achieve optimal developmental results, the JCIH recommends that all infants be screened by 1 month of age, receive audiologic confirmation by 3 months, and commence appropriate intervention by 6 months (1-3-6 timeline). In the absence of effective UNHS implementation, the mean age of detection remains approximately 14 months, and mild or unilateral hearing losses are often not diagnosed until school entry [18, 21]. An efficient UNHSP should demonstrate zero false negatives, ≤3% false positives, and referral rates ≤4%, alongside 95% population coverage and 95% follow-up compliance. These parameters are attainable using evoked otoacoustic emissions combined with automated auditory brainstem response (AABR) in a two-stage screening model, or AABR alone [21]. Both techniques are non-invasive, rapid, and easily performed, though mild or frequency-specific losses may occasionally escape detection [18].

2.7 The benefits of UNHSP

The benefits of implementing UNHSPs in developing countries are profound, particularly for improving the developmental trajectories of infants with permanent childhood hearing loss [22]. Auditory stimulation begins in utero and peaks by the sixth postnatal month, with the most rapid neural growth occurring within the first three months of life [22]. Undetected neonatal hearing loss adversely affects speech, language, academic achievement, and socio-emotional development, whereas early identification and intervention before six months are consistently associated with markedly better outcomes [8, 18]. Research demonstrates that infants diagnosed and rehabilitated before six months perform 20–40 percentile points higher on vocabulary, articulation, intelligibility, social adjustment, and behavioural scales than those diagnosed later [6, 23]. In the United States, the average cost of special education services for a child who is deaf or hard of hearing is USD 11,006 per year, while early detection and management can save approximately USD 400,000 per child in lifetime educational expenditure [24]. Evidence from the Colorado Newborn Screening Program shows that infants identified and treated by six months – except those with bilateral profound loss – can achieve age-appropriate language development comparable to peers with normal hearing [25]. Given the significant socio-economic burden and disability associated with PCEHL, early diagnosis and timely intervention are critical, particularly in developing contexts where affected children often receive no formal education and adults with hearing loss experience disproportionately high unemployment rates and under-employment [8, 26]. An effective UNHSP is therefore essential to altering the life-course outcomes of affected children.

2.8 Barriers to a UNHSP in resource-limited settings

2.8.1 Lack of infrastructure and equipment

Inadequate infrastructure and limited access to screening equipment represent major barriers to establishing NHSPs in resource-constrained environments. A controlled test environment is essential, ideally with ambient noise levels below 40 dB SPL, to ensure accurate results [18]. However, the cost of distortion product otoacoustic emission (DPOAE) and AABR devices is prohibitively high in countries where more than 60% of the population lives on less than USD 1.25 per day [27]. Consequently, program implementation depends heavily on government funding, which remains inadequate in many LMICs [28]. Although some authors have suggested the use of calibrated mechanical noisemakers to elicit behavioural responses as a low-cost alternative, such tools are only suitable for detecting severe-to-profound hearing loss and lack validation for mild-to-moderate impairments [29]. This limitation restricts their utility in remote areas where comprehensive physiologic screening is most needed, as all hearing losses exceeding 30 dB HL in either ear are classified by the WHO's International Classification of Functioning, Disability and Health for Children and Youth as potentially disabling [22].

2.8.2 Weak policies and legal framework

Weak policy direction and the absence of a supportive legal framework remain major obstacles to the institutionalisation of newborn hearing screening in LMICs. Although the WHO (2000) recommended that universal neonatal hearing screening be adopted wherever rehabilitation services are available, the first national policy statement did not appear until 2004. In Nigeria, the health-sector allocation represented only 3.4% of the national budget at that time and has risen modestly to about 5% as of 2024, still far below the Abuja Declaration target of 15% [27]. Persistent issues of under-financing, weak quality-assurance systems, loss to follow-up, and limited cost-effectiveness evaluations continue to undermine attempts to establish a functional national program [1].

2.8.3 Inadequate manpower and skilled personnel

A critical shortage of trained personnel – including audiologists, otolaryngologists, paediatricians, and other hearing-care professionals – poses a major impediment to UNHSP implementation in developing countries. Many

LMICs lack the financial capacity to train, recruit, and retain specialised staff [28]. Studies have demonstrated the feasibility of training non-specialist health workers for basic screening roles following structured training programs lasting two weeks to three months, offering a practical approach to workforce expansion in resource-limited settings [12, 29].

2.8.4 Low health budget

Inadequate health-care financing represents one of the fundamental constraints to implementing universal hearing screening in countries such as Nigeria. The national health budget – approximately ₦16 billion (compared with USD 23 trillion in the United States) – illustrates the disparity in fiscal capacity [28]. The high birth rate, coupled with severe resource shortages, renders large-scale nationwide screening unattainable in the short term. Except for HIV/AIDS screening, which benefits from international funding, child-health screening programs in Nigeria receive minimal domestic support [22]. Consequently, both private and public implementers must choose between universal and targeted models, often constrained to hospital-based or limited community-level interventions. At the policy level, decision-making is typically influenced by efficiency parameters such as cost per infant screened, cost per case detected, and follow-up performance [22].

2.8.5 Other contextual and individual factors

Beyond systemic barriers, several individual and sociocultural factors influence participation in hearing screening and rescreening activities. Evidence from pilot studies highlights low parental awareness, limited understanding of early intervention, transportation challenges, financial hardship, and cultural stigma associated with deafness as major deterrents [30]. Additional contributors include parental denial, illiteracy, superstitious beliefs, and negative attitudes towards medical screening [30]. Even in settings where programs are established, issues such as loss to follow-up, inadequate data management systems, inconsistent personnel training, high staff turnover, and the absence of standardised screening protocols persist, further undermining program effectiveness [31]. These personal and systemic barriers are surmountable, but there is a need for context-specific solutions as opposed to broad, generic measures.

2.9 Why a pilot study is needed?

To address these numerous barriers, the WHO recommends that each country undertake pilot studies to identify context-specific challenges and inform the design of an effective, sustainable UNHSP [32]. Such preliminary studies are essential for tailoring implementation strategies to local infrastructure, policy frameworks, and cultural realities. Moreover, establishing a UNHSP within every population is imperative because approximately 40% of infants with congenital hearing impairment present no identifiable risk factors or known aetiologies [26]. Consequently, targeted screening, which focuses on infants with recognisable perinatal clinical risks – such as birth asphyxia, congenital infections, exposure to ototoxic medications, hyperbilirubinemia, or chronic otitis media – inevitably misses a substantial proportion of affected infants [20]. By contrast, a universal screening approach ensures the early detection of both preventable and idiopathic cases, thereby enabling timely intervention and improved developmental outcomes [32].

This pilot study was necessary because, within the country's capital, there has been no prior UNHS initiative, and only a few targeted screening efforts have been reported in the literature. Previous studies conducted in other locations within the former capital were implemented through collaborations between the government, local private organisations, and international partners. However, those projects may not reflect the current realities of the post-COVID era, which has been characterised by economic instability, weakened health systems, and limited funding. Since then, a few isolated studies have been undertaken among well babies and high-risk infants, but none have specifically explored how resource-poor environments influence outcomes and compliance with recommended benchmarks for UNHSP.

Findings from this pilot study were expected to provide insight into the potential challenges and peculiarities that could affect the implementation of the 2018 National Policy and Strategic Plan for Ear and Hearing Care in the context of current resource limitations. The results also offer evidence-based guidance to inform policy review and strategic planning for the future scale-up of the UNHS program nationwide.

3. Methodology

3.1 Study design

The pilot study was conducted at Karshi General Hospital (KGH), Abuja Municipal Area Council. The hospital was purposively selected because it met predefined characteristics, including providing a suitable test environment and the availability of neonatal care services. KGH is a secondary-level facility and one of the 14 Federal Capital Territory Administration (FCTA) hospitals providing medical, surgical, obstetric, paediatric/neonatal, and emergency services. These hospitals also function as referral centres for surrounding primary healthcare facilities and private clinics.

3.2 Study duration and sampling

The study lasted nine months. Eligible participants were newborns aged ≤28 days, regardless of gestational age, who were delivered at or presented to KGH during the study period. Consecutive sampling of all eligible infants continued until the desired sample size was reached. Using the standard formula for populations <10,000, a minimum sample size of approximately 1,112 was calculated; allowing for 20% attrition increased this to 1,390. Therefore, the estimated sample size for the pilot study was 139. A total of 154 newborns were enrolled, but complete analyses were available for 132. Inclusion criteria required parental consent. Exclusion criteria included congenital malformation of the external ear or canal that prevented adequate probe sealing, ear discharge, complete canal occlusion by vernix, or severe otitis externa.

3.3 Screening method

The hearing screening followed a two-stage protocol. Each infant underwent DPOAE testing in both ears, immediately followed by AABR testing, regardless of the OAE outcome. Both procedures were performed using the Otoport Advance OAE + ABR device (Otodynamics Ltd., UK), which features an in-ear calibration process to compensate for variations in ear-canal size and provides optimal accuracy below 3 kHz. Each ear was assessed independently.

3.4 Training and equipment calibration

A graduate research assistant received training on equipment handling and maintenance, data recording from parental reports and hospital records, and participant follow-up procedures. The assistant also served as a chaperone and interpreter (Hausa language) to enhance communication and participant trust. The handheld screening device remained within its initial manufacturer-specified calibration period and was recalibrated weekly before use.

3.5 Data collection and screening procedure

Each infant first underwent an otoscopic examination using an Essentry SPEC v3® otoscope to confirm the patency of the external canal, the absence of debris or discharge, and the integrity of the tympanic membrane. Before testing, infants were fed and soothed to a light-sleep state; if breastfeeding was insufficient, expressed breast milk was given. Parents remained present throughout the testing. To minimise false-positive results, any ear yielding a 'refer' outcome was retested twice before confirmation.

For DPOAE, two continuous pure-tone stimuli with specified frequencies (f_1/f_2 = 75/70 dB SPL) and intensities (L_1/L_2 = 65/55 dB SPL) were delivered via insert earphones. An in-built microphone picks up the signals (emissions), and the result, either a pass (negative for hearing loss) or refer (positive for hearing loss), was determined based on the signal-to-noise ratio (SNR) at each test frequency. Responses with a signal-to-noise ratio ≥6 dB at ≥4 frequencies (1, 1.5, 2, and 4 kHz) constituted a PASS.

For AABR, electrodes were applied after skin preparation with abrasive gel: active (+) on the forehead, reference (–) on the cheek, and ground on the nape. Stimuli were 1000 Hz tone bursts at 35 dB SPL, presented at 85 Hz. Responses were automatically classified as PASS or REFER using waveform-template correlation (an in-built template constructed from responses from 30 neonates and optimised for infants 34 weeks to 6 weeks of age) and the Fsp statistical algorithm (a measure of the likelihood that a response is present). All tests occurred in a quiet room (Doctor's office) where the ambient noise level was below 40 dBA. Newborns were screened ≥24 hours after birth or before discharge.

3.6 Follow-up and diagnostic referral

Infants who failed DPOAE but passed AABR, suggestive of middle-ear pathology, received a one-week course of broad-spectrum antibiotics and were rescreened. Those who passed DPOAE but failed AABR were also rescreened after one week. Infants failing both tests in one or both ears after rescreening were referred to an otolaryngologist for comprehensive diagnostic evaluation.

3.7 Data analysis

Data were analysed using IBM SPSS Statistics v25.0. Tests of normality revealed a positively skewed distribution. Continuous variables (eg, age, birth weight, gestational age) were summarised as means ± standard deviation, compared using Student's t-test, and presented in tables and charts. Categorical variables were summarised as frequencies and percentages. McNemar's test was used to compare DPOAE and AABR outcomes for the same infants. A one-sample z-test for proportions was used to compare the observed rescreen return rate to a hypothetical 50% compliance. Wilson score intervals were computed for proportions to provide better coverage in small samples. Results should be interpreted cautiously, given the small pilot study sample size and high attrition. A p-value of <0.05 was considered statistically significant.

3.8 Ethical considerations

Written informed consent was obtained from each infant's parent or primary caregiver before enrolment. Confidentiality was maintained throughout the study, and screening results were disclosed only to parents. Ethical approval was granted by the Federal Capital Territory Health Research Ethics Committee (FCTHREC). Parents of infants who failed rescreening were counselled and referred to the Otolaryngology Department, National Hospital, Abuja, for confirmatory diagnostic testing.

4. Results

4.1 Overview of screening outcome

A total of 152 newborns were recruited, 92.4% of whom were born in the hospital, as shown in **Table 1**. Of these, 132 (85.7%) underwent DPOAE and AABR testing; 103 (78.0%) obtained a PASS on the initial DPOAE, while 29 (22.0%) were classified as REFER, as shown in **Table 2**. For AABR, 117 (88.6%) passed, and 15 (11.4%) were referred. Overall, 10 (7.6%) infants returned for rescreening: six for DPOAE only, one for AABR only, and three for both tests. On rescreening, four infants continued to fail DPOAE in one or both ears, whereas all AABR rescreens yielded PASS results.

4.2 Bivariate analysis

AABR achieved a significantly higher pass rate than DPOAE within the same infants (McNemar's test, $p < 0.05$), as shown in **Table 2**. The rescreen return rate was significantly lower than the benchmark of 50% ($p = 0.0035$), and dropout among referred infants was both large (73.7%) and imprecisely estimated (95% CI: 58.0%–85.0%).

4.3 Feasibility analysis of this pilot study

Feasibility across four domains, consistent with WHO and JCIH guidelines for screening programs [18, 32] – technical feasibility, operational feasibility, economic feasibility, and social acceptability – was assessed as follows:

Variable	Category	Frequency (*n*)	Percentage (%)	Mean ± SD
Sex	Male	69	52.3	
	Female	63	47.7	
Age at first screening (days)	–	–	–	8.48 ± 7.16
Age at re-screen (days)	–	–	–	28.50 ± 17.17
Gestational age (weeks)	<34	2	1.5	
	34–36 + 6 days	9	6.8	
	37–42	121	91.7	39.01 ± 1.66
Birth weight (kg)	1.5–2.49	21	15.9	
	2.5–3.99	100	75.8	
	≥ 4.0	11	8.3	3.08 ± 0.67
Term of birth	Term	121	91.7	
	Preterm	11	8.3	
Place of birth	Home	7	5.3	
	Hospital	122	92.4	
	Clinic	2	1.5	
	Others	1	0.8	
Rescreening status	Yes	10	7.6	
	No	122	92.4	
Referral status (any test)	Yes	38	28.8	
	No	94	71.2	

Table 1.
Sociodemographic and clinical characteristics of study participants (n = 132).

Screening test	Pass (*n*, %)	Refer (*n*, %)	Re-screened (*n*, %)	Referred for diagnostic test (*n*, %)	Mean age at test (days ± SD)
DPOAE	103 (78.0%)	29 (22.0%)	9 (6.8%)	4 (3.0%)	8.48 ± 7.16
AABR	117 (88.6%)	15 (11.4%)	4 (3.0%)	0 (0%)	8.48 ± 7.16

Table 2.
Screening outcomes.

4.3.1 Technical feasibility

Both the DPOAE and AABR were successfully implemented under local resource constraints. The Otoport Advance® device performed reliably throughout the study, and all screenings were completed without interruption, despite an unstable electricity supply. The average screening duration per infant (noted in logs as under 10 minutes) and the absence of equipment breakdowns support the technical operability of physiological screening in a low-resource environment. Statistically,

AABR achieved a higher pass rate (88.6%) than DPOAE (78.0%), and McNemar's test confirmed this difference was significant ($p = 0.022$), establishing AABR as the more robust option in noisy or uncontrolled test environments typical of hospitals.

4.3.2 Operational feasibility

The screening process was implemented by a single trained research assistant supervised by the principal investigator, demonstrating that minimal staff – when properly trained – can conduct neonatal hearing screening. Coverage was limited to 17.2% of eligible births (163/946), mainly due to staffing and resource constraints. Attrition totalled 19.8%, with a post-screen loss of 13.1% and a dropout rate of 73.7% among referrals. The rescreen return rate (26.3%) was significantly below the 50% benchmark ($p = 0.0035$), indicating that follow-up continuity is the main operational weakness.

4.3.3 Economic feasibility

Direct financial analysis was not performed; however, observed logistical adaptations (battery-operated device, printed proformas, local data storage) illustrate cost-efficiency measures applicable in low-resource settings. Given that screening time per infant was short and that a single device served over 130 cases, the cost per infant screened is likely to be low compared to the long-term cost of untreated childhood hearing loss. The significant AABR advantage (higher accuracy with a single test) may further reduce costs through fewer rescreens and false positives.

4.3.4 Social acceptability and cultural feasibility

Only 17.2% parental participation (163 of 946 mothers) reflects low initial acceptability, primarily due to limited awareness and understanding. Most families expressed willingness once informed, suggesting that low coverage resulted more from inadequate sensitisation than from cultural opposition. The involvement of a bilingual assistant improved participation and compliance among the Hausa-speaking mothers.

4.3.5 Diagnostic feasibility

Calculating and interpreting the sensitivity, specificity, positive predictive value (PPV), and negative predictive value (NPV) of the two-stage DPOAE + AABR protocol is a key element in evaluating the diagnostic feasibility and accuracy of a pilot screening program. However, it could not be done because none of the referrals presented themselves for diagnostic testing.

4.4 Rescreening and diagnostic follow-up challenges

All 132 participants completed both DPOAE and AABR screening. The overall REFER rate at the first screen was 28.8% (38 infants), affecting one or both ears. These infants were scheduled for rescreening; however, only 10 (26.3%) returned, corresponding to a dropout rate of 73.7% (the dropout rate was calculated as the proportion of infants referred for rescreening who did not return). The mean age at rescreening was 28.5 ± 17.2 days. Among those rescreened, the DPOAE rescreening rate was 31% (9 infants) and AABR 26.7% (4 infants). All rescreened passed except four (3.03%), who failed DPOAE and were referred for diagnostic evaluation at the nearest tertiary hospital equipped with full audiological and otologic services, approximately 43 km away. None of the referred infants presented for diagnostic follow-up.

4.5 Participant flow and logistical challenges

A total of 163 mothers or caregivers provided informed consent to participate; however, only 152 newborns were sampled, and after data cleaning, 132 were retained for analysis. The overall attrition rate was approximately 20%, consisting of pre-screen losses of 6.7% (11) and post-screen losses of 13.1% (20). All participants underwent both DPOAE and AABR screening at first contact, using a device equipped with a wireless data-transfer feature. Although the device could connect to a central server for efficient record-keeping, this function was not utilised due to the unavailability of computers, reliable internet connectivity, and stable network service. Nevertheless, partial data were stored locally on the screening device, which accommodated up to 250 patient entries and over 5,000 test results. Complementary information was collected using printed proformas that also served as a physical backup to prevent data loss. The Otoport Advance® device was handheld, portable, and battery-powered. It was fully charged before each screening session to prevent interruptions arising from power outages.

4.6 Human resource challenges

Most participants – 91 infants (68.9%) – were first screened within the first 10 days of life (**Figure 2**), a period that is often critical for both maternal recovery and neonatal adaptation, particularly regarding the establishment of lactation. Many mothers who opted for exclusive breastfeeding experienced initial difficulties due to limited professional lactation support. In the absence of such personnel, the principal investigator and the trained research assistant provided guidance and assisted mothers in expressing breastmilk to soothe irritable infants before screening. Because of budget constraints, only one research assistant could be trained; this individual undertook multiple responsibilities, including data entry, participant tracking, and follow-up of referrals. The facility lacked dedicated ear- or hearing-care professionals.

4.7 Individual and sociocultural challenges

A large majority of participants – 122 (92.4%) – were hospital-born. However, parental awareness and perception of newborn hearing screening were limited: Only 163 of 946 (17.2%) eligible parents provided consent, indicating low acceptance. Strategies implemented to improve participation included noticeboard communication and daily health-education sessions by healthcare staff. Professional interpreters were unavailable; therefore, the research assistant, fluent in Hausa, provided real-time translation for parents as required to overcome language barriers.

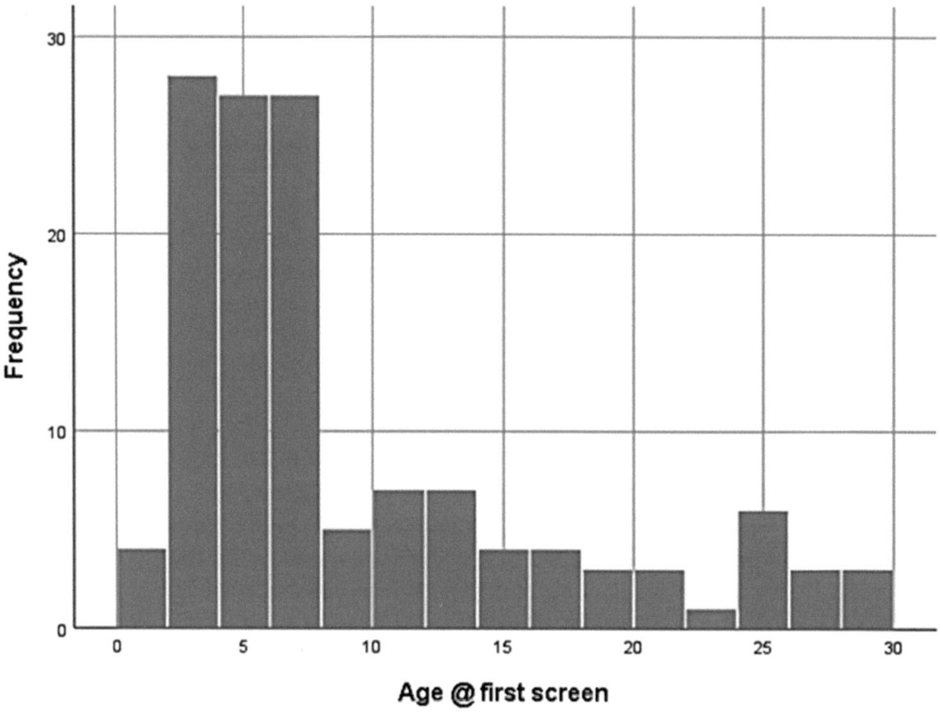

Figure 2.
Showing the age at first screen.

5. Discussion

5.1 Overview and context

Universal newborn hearing screening program in Nigeria, as with most developing countries, has remained at an infantile stage despite the efforts of individuals, stakeholders, and government agencies to initiate the program in line with global standards. This section provides an in-depth discussion of context-specific, immediate, and remote factors influencing the current state of UNHSP development and feasibility. Neonatal hearing screening is built on the principles of early detection, objective physiologic testing, high sensitivity and specificity, risk-factor monitoring, family-centred care, and integration into existing health systems – all aimed at ensuring optimal auditory, speech, language, and cognitive development in affected children [33].

5.2 Presentation of key findings

In this pilot study, the referral (REFER) rate in one or both ears following rescreen was 3.03% (mainly DPOAE), while the total referral rate for diagnostic hearing evaluation among infants in an urban community was 4.1% and 3.5% in a hospital-based study [11, 12]. These findings are comparable, although variations in study design, funding, screening protocol, and sample size may account for inherent differences. The high dropout rate observed here mirrors those reported in other LMICs, such as Pakistan, which recorded a 70% dropout rate attributed to financial hardship, poor transportation, limited awareness, sociocultural stigma, and parental denial of hearing loss [31]. A similarly high rescreen dropout rate (58.1%) was also reported in a tertiary facility in Ibadan, Nigeria [22].

5.3 Screening protocol and cost implications

The two-stage screening protocol adopted, DPOAE immediately followed by AABR, is widely recognised as the most precise, though also one of the most expensive, with a relatively high fail rate [34]. Nevertheless, the referral rate achieved in this study aligns with international standards of ≤4% for a viable screening program.

A major challenge encountered during this study was the lack of adequate funding – an essential foundation for implementing any UNHSP. Funds were required for the procurement of the screening device, staff training and deployment, infrastructure setup, follow-up and referral tracking, as well as communication with parents via calls or text reminders. Despite these limitations, cost–benefit analyses from published literature consistently demonstrate that newborn hearing screening yields substantial long-term benefits [28, 35–37]. Studies from developed countries indicate that universal physiological screening is more cost-effective than targeted screening or behavioural questionnaires [1].

Globally, unaddressed hearing loss imposes an estimated annual cost of 750 billion international dollars, including health-care expenditures (excluding hearing devices), educational support, productivity loss, and societal costs [8]. Early diagnosis and intervention reduce the need for special education, facilitate normal language development, and improve lifelong productivity. Even though detailed cost analyses are lacking in some LMICs [1, 38], existing evidence confirms that UNHSPs represent a sound societal investment [35].

A Lagos-based community screening program within immunisation clinics demonstrated greater cost-effectiveness than hospital-based screening for early detection of PCEHL [36]. However, critical considerations included transport accessibility, the proximity of diagnostic centres (≤5 km), and on-site screening to minimise loss to follow-up. Underlying yet overarching factors – economic downturn, global inflation, humanitarian crises, and weak socioeconomic policies – have further undermined the health systems and currencies of LMICs, diverting attention from this largely unapparent yet significant disability. To overcome these barriers, some authors recommend a programmatic approach where ear and hearing health are integrated into existing child-health initiatives such as school health programs, immunisation, prevention of mother-to-child transmission of HIV, maternal and child nutrition, and primary health-care outreach programs [39, 40].

5.4 Screening coverage and health-system factors

The screening coverage in this study was 17%, lower than other reports from the region. A 97% coverage was recorded in a community-based study at immunisation clinics in Lagos State, Nigeria, and this could be attributed to support provided by international partners, but the proportion of infants eligible from the total population could not be determined [41]. Although hospital-based studies may not capture population-wide trends due to variable health-service utilisation, hospital deliveries have risen to 49% compared with 25% in earlier national surveys [42, 43]. Only 3% of infants in this study were born outside the hospital, implying a strong potential for in-facility screening if properly implemented. The low coverage observed likely reflects economic hardship, ignorance of screening benefits, and geographic (rural) or infrastructural barriers [30]. Other contributory factors may include socio-political instability, cultural beliefs, and myths about deafness screening and diagnoses [44]. Environmental limitations, such as securing a quiet testing space, also posed challenges. In this study, the physician's consulting office in a relatively quiet section of the hospital was used, which, though functional, might have constrained coverage.

5.5 Operational efficiency and staffing

Depending on the device used, the average test duration for DPOAE is about 60 seconds, while AABR averages 10 minutes. Combining both within a single session in this study ensured that sensory, neural, and auditory neuropathy components were evaluated simultaneously, minimising false results and reducing dropout between stages. Each screening session required roughly 45 minutes per infant, accounting for all procedures, including otoscopy, feeding (including with EBM), and soothing.

Human-resource constraints limited the number of babies screened per day (approximately five) against a backdrop of weekly testing. With additional trained personnel, screening frequency and daily throughput could increase substantially. Although some feasibility studies have reported using trained non-specialists, each member of this study's small team – nurse, audiologist, paediatrician, and research assistant – played distinct roles vital to pre- and post-testing procedures, data integrity, and parental engagement. Even where non-specialists are trained as screeners, they still relied on the existing primary healthcare workers to educate parents on the value of the program [28, 45]. Thus, a robust, effective, and sustainable UNHSP should incorporate both approaches.

5.6 Timing of screening and attrition

The optimal window for screening was found to be within the first two weeks of life (days 2 to 10 in this study), ideally before discharge after caesarean delivery or during early immunisation or post-natal check-up visits, with higher chances of reduced referrals and loss to follow-up [2, 15, 46]. Screening beyond this period was difficult because most mothers did not return to the facility [2]. Early discharge after vaginal delivery (a common phenomenon in public hospitals in the country) further reduced in-hospital screening opportunities, as was reported in Singapore [47]. In one study, vaginal delivery was a significant predictor of loss to follow-up [48].

Attrition before screening reached 66% in comparable studies [49] and may stem from poor awareness of the benefits of early hearing detection. High post-screen dropout rates, often related to financial hardship [30], are further compounded by weak infrastructure, with few ear and hearing care specialists [38, 50] and long distances to tertiary diagnostic centres (up to 43 km in this study). Similar barriers have been documented in countries with low gross national income [33], where the impact of changes in the global economy, climate, health, and social services, particularly in the post-COVID era, may be more evident [3]. Such settings are characterised by delays in accessing diagnostic services and irregularities in the screening process [47].

5.7 Parental acceptance and sociocultural influences

Parental acceptance was low, contributing to limited coverage, despite the screening being provided free of charge. Some parents declined participation because they associated hearing screening with bad luck or spiritual connotations (jinx). To increase participation, health education and awareness campaigns were incorporated into routine hospital services, including antenatal, breastfeeding support, and postnatal clinics. Other measures reported in the literature – such as including hearing screening in post-delivery examinations or providing free transportation – significantly reduced default rates [48, 51].

Previous studies have linked low acceptance and default to misconceptions such as 'my baby can hear' (49.5%), 'no family history of hearing loss' (12.6%), or 'too costly' (10.8%) [47]. In similar settings with comparable default rates, reasons given were transportation difficulties (41%), lack of information or knowledge about the referral process (60%), and financial barriers (33%), while some expected a community health worker's visit to their homes [51]. Factors such as ignorance, illiteracy, superstition, and cultural myths about deafness remain widespread [38].

5.8 Comparative insights from high-resource settings

Unlike in high-income countries (HICs) with established UNHSPs and legislative backing, most LMICs lack standardised national protocols [31] and data management and tracking systems, which serve to reduce default and increase coverage [52]. However, even robust programs, such as those in Saudi Arabia, report challenges like loss to follow-up, inadequate data tracking, and inconsistent protocols [31]. These issues, while universal, are more pronounced in resource-limited settings where funding depends on government allocations rather than mixed public–private models [22, 28].

5.9 Unique insights from remote or low-resource contexts

Preventable causes of childhood hearing loss – such as chronic otitis media – are disproportionately higher in LMICs (75%) compared with HICs (49%) due to a lack of screening for the condition and appropriate treatment [8]. In this study, some infants who failed initial OAE screening passed after antibiotic therapy, indicating transient middle-ear pathology, while the few persistent failures likely represented sensory loss.

Because this was the first study of its kind in the region, communication in the local lingua franca (Hausa) proved essential for building trust and ensuring comprehension. Persistent misconceptions, cultural barriers, and poor socioeconomic conditions underscore the need for community participation, mass campaigns, and integration into existing primary health-care structures [28, 53]. Some studies have demonstrated successful integration into immunisation clinics, citing a reduction in loss to follow-up and higher coverage as benefits [38, 45]. However, a drawback was a higher age at first screen and re-screen, with potentially poor compliance with the 1-3-6 guideline.

5.10 Lessons learned from the pilot study

- The most effective screening window is within the first two weeks of life, ideally before discharge or during early postnatal visits.
- A two-stage DPOAE → AABR protocol provides comprehensive coverage of the auditory pathway, with minimal false positives or false negatives.
- Multidisciplinary collaboration – including nurses, lactation counsellors, obstetricians, paediatricians, audiologists, otolaryngologists, and social workers – is critical for sustainability.
- Increasing screening frequency (daily vs. weekly) can enhance coverage and reduce loss to follow-up.
- Sustained public education and awareness programs, particularly targeting rural women, are necessary to improve participation and compliance.

5.11 Implications for scaling-up UNHSP in LMICs

- Integration into primary health care (PHC) systems, as recommended by the WHO, will promote sustainability.
- Collaboration with local and international partners for funding, training, and technical support is crucial for building capacity and sustainable development.
- Establishing multiple screening units in high-population areas enhances cost-effectiveness and accessibility.
- Advocating for increased government health funding and reduced out-of-pocket expenditure will strengthen service delivery.
- Training non-specialist screeners on device use, data management, and patient engagement can expand coverage and continuity of care.
- Expanding the training curriculum for health and medical workers will increase ear and hearing care specialists.

5.12 Recommendations

i. Increase public awareness through community campaigns, mass media, and hospital-based health talks.

ii. Advocate for national legislation mandating UNHSP implementation at all levels of care.

iii. Develop standardised screening protocols and policies applicable across facilities.

iv. Foster international collaboration for funding and technical assistance.

v. Use integrated screening devices combining DPOAE and AABR for efficiency, flexibility, and adaptability.

vi. Establish digital data-tracking systems, ideally solar-powered, for follow-up and record management.

vii. Engage multidisciplinary teams, including non-specialist health staff, in hearing-screening delivery.

viii. Strengthen primary-health-care infrastructure to serve as a foundational platform for UNHSP implementation.

5.13 Research gaps

Further pilot qualitative or mixed-methods studies are needed to explore the sociocultural, logistical, and behavioural determinants of UNHS uptake and loss to follow-up in resource-limited environments.

6. Conclusion

Universal newborn hearing screening is a globally endorsed public-health measure for the early detection of PCEHL. Unaddressed hearing loss has profound developmental, educational, and socioeconomic consequences. This pilot study demonstrates that facility-based UNHSPs are feasible in resource-constrained settings using a two-stage DPOAE–AABR protocol. The approach achieved low referral rates consistent with international standards. A multidisciplinary, integrated, and well-funded strategy – implemented within the first two weeks of life – can significantly improve early detection and intervention outcomes in similar environments.

Acknowledgments

The authors express profuse gratitude to the Medical Director, Doctor Sanni Wilfred, and the entire management and staff of Karshi General Hospital for the support and access granted to use the facility's infrastructure throughout the period of this work. Contributions of the audiologist, Dr Adewumi Ojetoyinbo, to the conception and execution of this work are hereby acknowledged.

Conflict of interest

The authors declare no conflict of interest.

Nomenclature

AABR	Automated Auditory Brainstem Response
ABR	Auditory Brainstem Response

AIDS	Acquired Immunodeficiency Syndrome
CI	Confidence Interval
COVID-19	Coronavirus Disease 2019
dB	Decibel
dBA	A-weighted Decibel
dBHL	Decibel Hearing Level
DPOAE	Distortion Product Otoacoustic Emission
EBM	Expressed Breast Milk
EHDI	Early Hearing Detection and Intervention
ENT	Ear, Nose and Throat
FCT	Federal Capital Territory
FCTA	Federal Capital Territory Administration
Fsp	Statistical test ratio used in ABR detection algorithms
HICs	High-Income Countries
HREC	Health Research Ethics Committee
Hz	Hertz (cycles per second)
IBM	International Business Machines Corporation
JCIH	Joint Committee on Infant Hearing
KGH	Karshi General Hospital
LMICs	Low- and Middle-Income Countries
n	Sample size or number of participants
NPV	Negative Predictive Value
OAE	Otoacoustic Emission
PCEHL	Permanent Congenital Early-Onset Hearing Loss
PCHI	Permanent Childhood Hearing Impairment
PCHL	Permanent Congenital Hearing Loss
PHC	Primary Health Care
PPV	Positive Predictive Value
P-value	Probability value indicating statistical significance.
SD	Standard Deviation
SNR	Signal-to-Noise Ratio
SPL	Sound Pressure Level
SPSS	Statistical Package for the Social Sciences
UNHS	Universal newborn hearing screening
UNHSP	Universal newborn hearing screening program
WHO	World Health Organization

Author details

Oyinwola Oluwafisayo[1*], Ozioko Obialunamma[2] and Oluwasola Timothy[3]

1 Karshi General Hospital, Abuja, Nigeria

2 National Hospital, Abuja, Nigeria

3 University College Hospital, Ibadan, Nigeria

*Address all correspondence to: fisayooyinwola@gmail.com

References

[1] World Health Organization. Newborn and infant hearing screening: Current issues and guiding principles for action [Internet]. 2009. Available from: https://iris.who.int/server/api/core/bitstreams/afa7b52d-143a-4077-b2de-adf0d156e936/content [Accessed: 2025-October-11]

[2] Olusanya BO, Luxon LM, Wirz SL. Benefits and challenges of newborn hearing screening for developing countries. International Journal of Pediatric Otorhinolaryngology. 2004;**68**:287–305. DOI: 10.1016/S0165-5876(03)00404-X

[3] Edeh HC, Nnamani AU, Ozor JO. Effect of COVID-19 on catastrophic medical spending and forgone care in Nigeria. Economies. 2025;**13**:116. DOI: 10.3390/economies13050116

[4] Okhakhu AI, Ibekwe TS, Sadoh AS, Ogisi FO. Neonatal hearing screening in Benin City. International Journal of Pediatric Otorhinolaryngology. 2010;**74**:1323–1326. DOI: 10.1016/j.ijporl.2010.08.017

[5] Abdullahi A, Shofoluwe NA, Abubakar A, Sandabe MB, Garandawa HI, Babatunde MI, et al. Neonatal hearing screening with otoacoustic emission among normal babies in a northeastern Nigerian hospital. Journal of West African College of Surgeons. 2021;**11**:11

[6] World Health Organization. Childhood hearing loss: Strategies for prevention and care [Internet]. 2016. Available from: https://apps.who.int/iris/bitstream/handle/10665/204632/9789241510325_eng.pdf?sequence=1&isAllowed=y [Accessed: 2025-May-22]

[7] Plack CJ. The Sense of Hearing. 3rd ed. New York: Taylor & Francis; 2018. p. 338. DOI: 10.4324/9781315208145

[8] World Health Organization. Deafness and hearing loss [Internet]. 2017. Available from: https://www.who.int/news-room/fact-sheets/detail/deafness-and-hearing-loss [Accessed: 2025-January-11]

[9] Hepper PG, Shahidullah BS. Development of fetal hearing. Archives of Disease in Childhood: Fetal and Neonatal Edition. 1994;**71**:F81–F87. DOI: 10.1136/fn.71.2.F81

[10] World Health Organization. Global spending on health: Emerging from the pandemic [Internet]. 2024. Available from: https://iris.who.int/server/api/core/bitstreams/6a22149b-17d5-4afb-a89b-14a3e8c12442/content#page=1.00&gsr=0 [Accessed: 2025-October-6]

[11] Olusanya BO, Wirz SL, Luxon LM. Community-based infant hearing screening for early detection of permanent hearing loss in Lagos, Nigeria: A cross-sectional study. Bulletin of the World Health Organization. 2008;**86**:956–963. DOI: 10.2471/BLT.07.050005

[12] Olusanya BO, Wirz SL, Luxon LM. Hospital-based universal newborn hearing screening for early detection of permanent congenital hearing loss in Lagos, Nigeria. International Journal of Pediatric Otorhinolaryngology. 2008;**72**:991–1001. DOI: 10.1016/j.ijporl.2008.03.004

[13] Federal Ministry of Health (Nigeria). National policy and strategic plan for ear and hearing care 2019–2013 [Internet]. 2019. Available from: https://

www.policyvault.africa/policy/nationa l-policy-and-strategic-plan-for-ear-and -hearing-care-2019-2013/ [Accessed: 2025-September-16]

[14] Labaeka AA, Tongo OO, Ogunbosi BO, Fasunla JA. Prevalence of hearing impairment among high-risk newborns in Ibadan, Nigeria. Front Pediatr. 2018;**6**:194. DOI: 10.3389/fped. 2018.00194

[15] Akinola MD, Onakoya PA, Tongo O, Lasisi AO. Neonatal hearing screening using transient evoked otoacoustic emission in a sub-urban population in Nigeria. International Journal of Otolaryngology and Head and Neck Surgery. 2014;**3**:205–211. DOI: 10.4236/ijohns.2014.34038

[16] Lasisi AO, Onakoya PA, Lasisi TJ, Akinola MD, Tongo O. Neonatal hearing screening in a rural/sub-urban community in Nigeria, sub-Saharan Africa–A preliminary report. International Journal of Pediatric Otorhinolaryngology. 2014;**78**:1452–1455. DOI: 10.1016/j.ijporl.2014.06.003

[17] Oyinwola OI, Mukhtar-Yola M, Olusesi AD, Oluwasola TA. Automated ABR screening for hearing loss and its clinical determinants among newborns with hyperbilirubinemia in National Hospital, Abuja, Nigeria. Nigerian Journal of Clinical Practice. 2023;**26**:1249–1256. DOI: 10.4103/njcp.njcp_449_22

[18] American Speech-Language-Hearing Association, Joint Committee on Infant Hearing. Year 2007 position statement: Principles and guidelines for early hearing detection and intervention [Internet]. 2007. Available from: www .asha.org/policy [Accessed: 2025-May-9]

[19] Olusanya BO, Davies AC, Hoffman HJ. Hearing loss grades and the International classification of functioning, disability and health. Bulletin of the World Health Organization. 2019;**97**:725–728. DOI: 10.2471/BLT.19.230367

[20] World Health Organization. WHO global estimates on prevalence of hearing loss: Mortality and burden of diseases and prevention of blindness and deafness [Internet]. 2012. Available from: https://www.who.int/pbd/deaf ness/WHO_GE_HL.pdf?ua=1 [Accessed: 2025-February-16]

[21] American Academy of Pediatrics. Newborn and infant hearing loss: detection and intervention. Pediatrics. 1999;**103**:527–530. DOI: 10.1542/ peds.103.2.527

[22] Olusanya BO. Neonatal hearing screening and intervention in resource-limited settings: An overview. Archives of Disease in Childhood. 2012;**97**:654–659. DOI: 10.1136/archdis child-2012-301786

[23] Jose O, Sreelatha PR, Nath RR. Assessment of hearing impairment using brainstem evoked response audiometry (BERA) in neonates with various otonoxious risk factors. IOSR Journal of Dental and Medical Sciences. 2017;**16**:25–33. DOI: 10.9790/0853-1603022533

[24] Centers for Disease Control and Prevention. Screening and diagnosis: Hearing loss [Internet]. 2016. Available from: https://www.cdc.gov/ncbddd/hea ringloss/screening.html [Accessed: 2025-April-22]

[25] Yoshinaga-Itano C, Coulter BA, Thomson MA. The Colorado newborn hearing screening project: Effects on speech and language development for children with hearing loss. Journal of

Perinatology. 2000;**20**:S132–7. DOI: 10.1038/sj.jp.7210381

[26] Olusanya BO, Newton VE. Global burden of childhood hearing impairment and disease control priorities for developing countries. The Lancet. 2007;**369**:1314–1317. DOI: 10.1016/S0140-6736(07)60602-3

[27] Federal Ministry of Health (Nigeria). The state of the health of the nation report 2024 [Internet]. 2024. Available from: https://fmohconnect.gov.ng/wp-content/uploads/2025/05/The-State-of-the-Health-of-the-Nation-Report-2024.pdf#page=63.08 [Accessed: 2025-October-31]

[28] Olusanya BO, Swanepoel DW, Chapchap MJ, Castillo S, Habib H, Mukari SZ, et al. Progress towards early detection services for infants with hearing loss in developing countries. BMC Health Services Research. 2007;**7**:14

[29] Ramesh A, Jagdish C, Nagapoorinima M, Rao PNS, Ramakrishnan AG, Thomas GC, et al. Low-cost calibrated mechanical noisemaker for hearing screening. Indian Journal of Medical Research. 2012;**135**:182–188

[30] Pyarali M, Akhtar S, Adeel M, Mallick SA, Uneeb SN, Aslam A. Neonatal hearing screening program and challenges faced by the developing country: A tertiary care hospital experience. Journal of the Pakistan Medical Association. 2023;**73**:6264. DOI: 10.47391/JPMA.6264

[31] Alanazi AA, Nicholson N. Challenges of newborn hearing screening programs in Saudi Arabia: A systematic review. Audiology Research. 2025;**15**:34. DOI: 10.3390/audiolres15020034

[32] World Health Organization. World report on hearing [Internet]. 2021. Available from: https://www.who.int/publications/i/item/9789240020481 [Accessed: 2025-October-31]

[33] Bussé AML, Hoeve HLJ, Nasserinejad K, Mackey AR, Simonsz HJ, Goedegebure A. Prevalence of permanent neonatal hearing impairment: Systematic review and Bayesian meta-analysis. International Journal of Audiology. 2020;**59**:475–485. DOI: 10.1080/14992027.2020.1716087

[34] Wroblewska-Seniuk KE, Dabrowski P, Szyfter W, Mazela J. Universal newborn hearing screening: Methods and results, obstacles, and benefits. Pediatric Research. 2017;**81**:415–422. DOI: 10.1038/pr2016250

[35] Gorga MP, Neely ST. Cost-effectiveness and test-performance factors in relation to universal newborn hearing screening. Mental Retardation and Developmental Disabilities Research Reviews. 2003;**9**:103–108. DOI: 10.1002/mrdd.10066

[36] Olusanya BO, Emokpae A, Renner JK, Wirz SL. Costs and performance of early hearing detection programmes in Lagos, Nigeria. Transactions of the Royal Society of Tropical Medicine and Hygiene. 2009;**103**:179–186. DOI: 10.1016/j.trstmh.2008.07.001

[37] Colgan S, Lutman ME, Kitterick PT, Charnock T, Parker Z, Fielder R, et al. The cost-effectiveness of universal newborn screening for bilateral permanent congenital hearing

impairment: Systematic review. Health Technology Assessment. 2012;**16**:1–231

[38] Olusanya BO. Priorities for early hearing detection and intervention in sub-Saharan Africa. International Journal of Audiology. 2008;**47**:S3–13. DOI: 10.1080/14992020802287143

[39] Olusanya BO, Luxon LM, Wirz SL. Screening for early childhood hearing loss in Nigeria. Journal of Medical Screening. 2005;**12**:115–8. DOI: 10.1258/0969141054855274

[40] Sebothoma B, Khoza-Shangase K. Programmatic approach to hearing health in low- and middle-income countries. The Hearing Journal. 2023;**76**:36–42. DOI: 10.1097/01.HJ.0000921632.79554.71

[41] Olusanya BO, Ebuehi OM, Somefun AO. Universal infant hearing screening programme in a community with predominant non-hospital births: A three-year experience. Journal of Epidemiology and Community Health. 2009;**63**:481–487. DOI: 10.1136/jech.2008.082784

[42] United Nations Children's Fund (UNICEF). The state of the world's children 2024 statistical compendium [Internet]. 2024. Available from: https://data.unicef.org/resources/sowc-2024/ [Accessed: 2025-October-24]

[43] National Population Commission (Nigeria), ICF International. Nigeria Demographic and Health Survey 2018 [Internet]. 2019. Available from: www.DHSprogram.com [Accessed: 2025-January-2]

[44] Kiyaga NB, Moores DF. Deafness in Sub-Saharan Africa. American Annals of the Deaf. 2003;**148**:18–24. DOI: 10.1353/aad.2003.0004

[45] Health Professions Council of South Africa, Professional Board for Speech, Language and Hearing Professions. Early hearing detection and intervention programmes in South Africa: Position statement [Internet]. 2007. Available from: https://www.hpcsa.co.za/Uploads/editor/UserFiles/downloads/speech/early_hearing_detection_statement.pdf [Accessed: 2018-May-9]

[46] Mackey AR, Busse AML, Del Vecchio V, Maki-Torkko E, Uhlen IM. Protocol and programme factors associated with referral and loss to follow-up from newborn hearing screening: A systematic review. International Journal of Pediatric Otorhinolaryngology. 2022;**162**:111342. DOI: 10.1016/j.ijporl.2022.111342

[47] Low W, Pang K, Ho L, Lim S. Universal newborn hearing screening in Singapore: The need, implementation and challenges. Annals of the Academy of Medicine, Singapore. 2005;**34**:301–306. DOI: 10.47102/annals-aam/2005-0039

[48] Olusanya BO. Follow-up default in a hospital-based universal newborn hearing screening programme in a low-income country. Child: Care, Health and Development. 2009;**35**:190–198. DOI: 10.1111/j.1365-2214.2008.00923.x

[49] Jacob J, Kurien M, Sindhusha K, Kumar P, Krishnan L. Challenges of universal newborn hearing screening in a developing country: A double-edged sword. Indian Journal of Otolaryngology and Head and Neck Surgery. 2022;**74**:395–401. DOI: 10.1007/s12070-020-02170-8

[50] Majid AHA, Ismail AI, Ameen A, Musibau HO. Universal Newborn hearing screening programme in

Nigeria: Overview and emerging issues [Internet]. 2018. Available from: https://uilspace.unilorin.edu.ng/items/e6c18845-14e4-474a- 934e-fb11a7c22c10 [Accessed: 2020-January-02]

[51] Bright T, Mulwafu W, Thindwa R, Zuurmond M, Polack S. Reasons for low uptake of referrals to ear and hearing services for children in Malawi. PLoS One. 2017;**12**:e0188703. DOI: 10.1371/journal.pone.0188703

[52] Alanazi AA. Referral and lost to system rates of two newborn hearing screening programs in Saudi Arabia. International Journal of Neonatal Screening. 2020;**6**: p. 50 DOI: 10.3390/ijns6030050

[53] Federal Ministry of Health (NG). National Health Policy 2016 [Internet]. 2016. Available from: https://extranet.who.int/countryplanningcycles/sites/default/files/planning_cycle_repository/nigeria/draft_nigeria_national_health_policy_final_december_fmoh_edited.pdf [Accessed: 2025-September-16]

Section 2

Etiology and Pathophysiological Foundations

Chapter 2

Hearing Loss and Infectious Diseases

Milaine Dominici Sanfins, Daniela Gil and Piotr Henryk Skarzynski

Abstract

Hearing loss is a significant sequelae of many infectious diseases, both congenital and acquired, with a direct impact on communication and development. Damage to the auditory system is multifactorial and can occur directly, such as from inflammation and oxidative stress in the inner ear, or indirectly, such as from opportunistic infection or ototoxicity from drug treatments. Cytomegalovirus (CMV) and rubella are notorious causes of congenital hearing loss in children, while bacterial meningitis is one of the leading causes of acquired deafness in childhood. Other pathogens, such as measles, mumps, and HIV viruses, give rise to characteristic audiological profiles, with HIV in particular contributing to drug ototoxicity. COVID-19 has emerged as a new risk factor, with cochlear and central damage still under investigation. Given the complex nature of infection-related hearing loss, early detection and intervention are crucial. Optimal management requires a multidisciplinary approach involving infectious disease specialists, audiologists, and neurologists, with the aim of accurate diagnosis and effective rehabilitation of affected children. This chapter highlights the need to strengthen public health policies, with a focus on expanding vaccination coverage, implementing universal audiological screening programs, and continuously monitoring children at risk. Awareness of the auditory manifestations of infections is essential to ensure that a child's hearing is preserved and their development continues unimpaired.

Keywords: hearing loss, child development, infectious diseases, virus, hearing tests, auditory perception

1. Introduction

Hearing loss, especially sensorineural hearing loss, deriving from damage to the inner ear and/or auditory nerve, can significantly compromise a child's communication ability.

Some viral diseases, many of which are quite common during childhood and adolescence, can affect the auditory system both peripherally and centrally. In addition, some diseases, when contracted during pregnancy, can affect fetal development and consequently hearing. In fact, infectious diseases are major causes of both congenital and acquired hearing loss.

Looking first at the periphery, viruses can reach the inner ear through the bloodstream and lead to the accumulation of reactive oxygen species (ROS), which, in turn, can cause oxidative stress and subsequent cell death. If the hair cells of the inner ear are injured, this will lead to permanent and irreversible hearing loss.

To identify peripheral hearing loss, pure-tone audiometry by air conduction continues to be the gold standard. Thus, in cases of virus infection, a hearing threshold test is mandatory. In order to minimize damage, diagnosis and intervention should be carried out as early as possible.

In this chapter, we address the main infections that can compromise hearing, and, whenever possible, the audiological characteristics associated with each condition are listed.

2. Infectiology: Infectious diseases

Infectious diseases or infectiology, is a field of medicine that consists of four basic strands: (i) the effective prevention of infectious diseases, (ii) the accurate diagnosis of these diseases, (iii) the appropriate treatment of affected patients, and (iv) the search for a cure for conditions related to major infections.

Infectiology fundamentally protects public health, fighting microbiological threats that are continually emerging. In addition, it is central to the control of infections that occur within hospitals and is constantly seeking ways of preventing outbreaks of epidemics.

Currently, this science is facing a major global challenge in the form of antimicrobial resistance, which presents a global threat to public health. Recently, the role of infectious disease specialists has been put to the test, especially as a result of the emergence of COVID-19. There are also diseases such as Zika virus and Ebola that call for rapid and effective intervention.

As early as 2007, the WHO warned of the accelerated spread of viral diseases and the emergence of new infectious agents. The emergence and persistence of new pathogens constitute a continuous biological race, and the adaptive nature of new diseases and the constant search for new prevention and treatment strategies have become major pillars of modern medicine.

By definition, infectious diseases are disorders caused by organisms, mostly microscopic, that can be transmitted directly or indirectly between people or from infected animals to humans. The main etiological agents studied in infectious diseases include:

- **Viruses:** These acellular life forms are obligate intracellular parasites, requiring host cells to reproduce. They cause a wide range of diseases, such as COVID-19, influenza (flu), HIV/AIDS, Ebola, dengue, hepatitis, and measles [1–5].

- **Bacteria:** These single-celled microorganisms are prokaryotes that can be either pathogenic or, in many cases, beneficial (such as the components of the gut microbiota that aid digestion and protect us against pathogens). Examples of bacterial diseases include tuberculosis, salmonellosis, impetigo, cellulitis, syphilis, and leptospirosis. Bacterial resistance to antibiotics is a growing problem of great concern [6].

- **Fungi:** These are eukaryotic organisms that can cause superficial or systemic infections, the latter being of particular concern in immunocompromised individuals. Common examples include athlete's foot, candidiasis (yeast), ringworm, onychomycosis, and thrush [6].

- **Protozoa:** These are single-celled parasites that cause diseases such as malaria, toxoplasmosis, leishmaniasis, and amoebiasis [6].

- **Other parasites (helminths and ectoparasites):** These include worms, such as those that cause schistosomiasis and Chagas disease, and ectoparasites, such as lice and scabies [6].

When these agents overcome the body's natural defenses, they can multiply and disrupt normal physiological functions, leading to a wide spectrum of clinical manifestations, including alterations in the peripheral and central auditory systems [7].

3. The effect of infectious diseases on the auditory system

The human auditory system is a complex and highly specialized structure and is functionally and anatomically divided into peripheral and central components, which work together to capture, detect, process, and interpret sound.

Infectious diseases are a significant burden on global health, and they impose a considerable and often underestimated impact on hearing health. For children and adolescents, infections are important and often preventable causes of hearing loss, a challenge that is more pronounced in low- and middle-income countries [8–10].

Flawless functioning of the auditory system is needed for full neurocognitive and social development, especially in children, where language acquisition and educational progress depend directly on good hearing. Hearing loss, which is a common sequelae of a number of infections, can have life-long implications, impairing quality of life and full development, as well as costing the state financially.

In this context, early detection and intervention for hearing loss, especially in the pediatric population, are important for mitigating possible sequelae. Difficulties associated with these infections can arise as soon as a disease is acquired and even persist for years afterward [11].

There is also a need for awareness campaigns among the general population, especially for women of childbearing age, about the importance of immunization against infectious diseases. Immunization provides additional protection against sexually transmitted diseases, noting that syphilis, in vertical transmission, can have devastating effects on a child's development.

3.1 Auditory manifestations of specific viral infections

Viral infections represent a wide category of pathogens with the ability to affect the auditory system in various ways, from direct damage to cochlear structures to the induction of systemic inflammatory responses – or even as a result of ototoxic treatments.

3.1.1 Cytomegalovirus (CMV)

Cytomegalovirus (CMV) is a congenital infection that is a major risk indicator for sensorineural hearing loss. The pathogenic agent is the virus *Herpesviridae*. CMV is one of the infections included in the TORCH acronym [Toxoplasmosis, Others (Zika, HIV, Chickenpox, Parvovirus, Syphilis), Rubella, Cytomegalovirus, and Herpes]. In developed countries, congenital cytomegalovirus is the major cause of sensorineural hearing loss of non-genetic origin [12].

CMV is ubiquitous, with no seasonal variations, and is relatively common in women of childbearing age. It is an infectious disease that can be transmitted both horizontally – through contact with bodily fluids, such as saliva, urine, tears, and genital secretions – and vertically through the placenta, birth canal, or breastfeeding. The risk of vertical transmission increases with gestational age, being approximately 20% in the first trimester and 75% in the third. For some reason, the severity of CMV sequelae is lower the higher the gestational age. When acquired postnatally, CMV is not a direct cause of hearing loss. Thus, the focus remains on the pediatric population and its susceptibility to congenital CMV [13]. The disease symptoms are the following:

- Often asymptomatic at birth
- Hepatosplenomegaly
- Petechiae
- Anaemia
- Leucopenia
- Chorioretinitis
- Hypotonia
- Brain atrophy
- Periventricular cysts
- Microcephaly
- Delay in psychomotor development
- Seizures.

Infection causes dysfunction of the stria vascularis, labyrinthitis, glial cytotoxicity, lesions in the organ of Corti and the cochlear ganglion, as well as alterations in the development of the inner ear. Hearing loss from CMV can compromise children at birth, whether they have symptoms or not, reinforcing the need for continual audiological monitoring if the serology is positive. Hearing loss can be congenital or late-onset. This follow-up should continue until the age of 6.

The characteristics of hearing loss usually follow the following pattern:

- Neurosensory type
- Variable degree (mild to profound)
- Unilateral or bilateral involvement
- Symmetrical or asymmetrical
- Variable and/or progressive.

Importantly, CMV is one of the most common causes of unilateral hearing loss and can be a clear indicator for unilateral cochlear implantation in a child due to the risk of progressive hearing loss in the better ear. A vaccine against CMV is a dire public health need; originally promised in the 1970s, a vaccine is currently in phase 3 studies and offers great hope for prophylaxis against CMV infection.

3.1.2 Toxoplasmosis

Congenital toxoplasmosis is an infection that occurs during pregnancy and is often linked to women from low- or middle-income economic classes [12]. The pathogen is the parasite, *Toxoplasma gondii,* found in contaminated water or food. Vertical transmission of the infection from mother to fetus can lead to the baby's death a few days after birth. Based on infected live births, 35% develop neurological diseases, 80% have eye problems, and about 40% have hearing loss. The pathophysiology of hearing loss remains unclear [14], although one hypothesis is that it is a postnatal inflammatory response. If true, then treatment with antimicrobials and antibiotics in the first week of life may prevent hearing loss [15].

The symptoms of the disease are:

- Prematurity
- Retarded intrauterine growth
- Jaundice
- Myocarditis
- Pneumonite
- Rash
- Hepatosplenomegaly
- Chorioretinitis

- Hydrocephalus
- Intracranial calcifications
- Seizures
- Microcephaly
- Asymptomatic at birth (common).

Manifestations can appear at different stages of development, and hearing loss may persist despite treatment. The disease causes widespread neurological damage that impacts sensory, visual, and auditory pathways. The characteristics of hearing loss usually follow the following pattern:

- Sensorineural or conductive
- Variable degree (mild to profound)
- Unilateral or bilateral
- Symmetrical or asymmetrical.

Incidentally, toxoplasmosis affects not only the peripheral auditory pathway but can also alter central auditory pathways as well. Since toxoplasmosis is a major global public health problem, patients with the condition should be monitored so that the impacts resulting from this infection can be limited [14].

3.1.3 Congenital/acquired syphilis

Acquired syphilis is a sexually transmitted infection (STI) resulting from sexual intercourse (vaginal, oral, or anal) without protection. It can exhibit several clinical manifestations at different stages, evident as primary, secondary, latent, or tertiary syphilis. The stages refer to the time of onset of symptoms, and in the tertiary stage, symptoms can appear decades after infection [12].

Congenital syphilis, on the other hand, occurs through transmission from the infected mother to the baby during pregnancy or at the time of delivery. The pathogenic agent is the bacterium, *Treponema pallidum*. WHO data from 2017 indicate that, for 37 of the 83 countries for which data were available, the incidence of syphilis in pregnant women was as high as 1% [15]. The symptoms of the disease are:

Congenital

- Most cases are asymptomatic at birth
- Maculopapular exanthem
- Papular lesions

- Bullous vesicle eruptions
- Generalized lymphodenopathy
- Hepatosplenomegaly
- Hydrocephalus
- Intellectual disability
- Sensorineural hearing loss.

Acquired

- Aortic disease
- Meningitis
- Genital ulcers
- Skin lesions
- Lymphodenopathy
- Neurological syndromes.

Hearing loss in congenital syphilis is irreversible. It can cause damage to the central nervous system or sensory pathways, such as those in the auditory system. In congenital syphilis, the pathophysiology of hearing loss involves extreme degeneration of the organ of Corti and the spiral ganglion, as well as labyrinthine hemorrhage and fibrin accumulation. The characteristics of hearing loss usually follow the following pattern:

- Neurosensory type
- Variable degree (moderate to severe)
- Unilateral or bilateral
- Symmetrical or asymmetrical
- Sudden or progressive
- Irreversible
- If progressive, it starts at high frequencies.

Studies indicate that syphilis is more frequent among younger pregnant women with low education, and there is a greater number of infected individuals in emerging countries. In some countries, the reemergence of congenital syphilis is known, which may be due to social vulnerabilities and economic inequalities. To reduce the number of cases, education campaigns on sexual protection methods, as well as vaccination campaigns, are needed.

Syphilis responds very well to treatment with penicillin, which is the treatment of choice. Treatment of mothers infected during pregnancy significantly reduces the chance of congenital syphilis and is therefore a priority from the point of view of public health.

3.1.4 HIV

Acquired immunodeficiency syndrome (AIDS) is an infectious disease transmitted by the Human Immunodeficiency Virus (HIV), which attacks the immune system, impairing its ability to defend the body against disease.

The symptoms of the pathology involve:

- Fever
- Fatigue
- Rash
- Headache
- Muscle and joint pain
- Sore throat
- Mouth ulcers
- Swollen lymph nodes
- Night sweats
- Diarrhea and weight loss.

The prevalence of hearing loss in individuals with HIV is notably higher than in the general population, evidencing the need for specialized care. Hearing loss in people with HIV/AIDS is not the result of a single cause but rather the manifestation of a complex, multifactorial interaction between the virus itself, opportunistic infections, and the effects of medications [16–19].

HIV exhibits a marked neurotropism, with the ability to penetrate and affect the central nervous system (CNS) in the early stages of infection. This viral involvement can cause direct damage to the auditory pathways, both peripheral and central, including the cochlear nerve.

Hearing damage can occur in three ways:

(i) Direct effect of the virus on the auditory system: The HIV virus itself can cause direct damage to the structures of the inner ear, leading to inflammation and degeneration of hair cells, which are essential for hearing. This viral damage can result in sensorineural hearing loss, which is one of the most common types of hearing loss in HIV patients. In addition, the virus can cause neuropathy, affecting the auditory nerve and impairing the transmission of sound signals to the brain.

(ii) Opportunistic infections: Because HIV weakens the immune system, people with the virus become more susceptible to opportunistic infections that can affect the ear. Some of the most common infections that cause hearing problems include the following. Chronic otitis media (persistent middle ear infections); Meningitis (inflammation of the membranes covering the brain and spinal cord, which can affect the auditory nerve); Herpes virus and cytomegalovirus (CMV) (viruses that can cause inflammation and damage to the inner ear). These infections can lead to conductive hearing loss (due to middle ear problems) or sensorineural hearing loss (affecting the cochlea).

(iii) Ototoxic medications: Although antiretroviral therapy is essential for the treatment of HIV, some medications, both older and current, can be ototoxic (that is, harmful to the ear). In addition, some medications used to treat opportunistic infections, such as certain antibiotics, can also cause hearing loss.

Otitis media is frequently identified as a cause of ear infections in HIV-positive patients, as well as otitis media with effusion. The hearing loss usually follows the following pattern:

- Conductive, sensorineural, or mixed type
- Variable degree (moderate to severe)
- Unilateral or bilateral
- Symmetrical or asymmetrical
- Sudden or progressive
- Tinnitus
- Vertigo
- Earache.

In the case of patients with HIV, regular audiological evaluation is important, and if alterations are found, auditory rehabilitation should be implemented. It is necessary to monitor patients to control the severity of HIV and prevent hearing complications.

3.1.5 Rubella

Rubella is an acute rash disease caused by the rubella virus, which belongs to the genus *Rubivirus* of the Togaviridae family [12, 20, 21]. The main route of transmission relevant to hearing loss is transplacental, from mother to fetus, resulting in Congenital Rubella Syndrome (CRS). Postnatal transmission occurs predominantly through direct contact with droplets of nasopharyngeal secretions from infected individuals. The symptoms of the disease are:

In pregnant women

- Mild fever
- Conjunctivitis
- Lymphadenopathy
- Rash
- It can be asymptomatic.

In fetuses and infants

- Microcephaly
- Meningoencephalitis
- Congenital cataract
- Retinopathy
- Heart defects
- Hepatosplenomegaly
- Bone radiolucences.

There is no specific treatment model. In newborns, the virus can be present for more than a year after infection and is more contagious in the first months of life [20, 21].

Hearing loss is one of the most frequent anomalies and often the earliest symptom of CRS. Hearing loss is permanent, even after treatment [22]. Hearing alterations result from direct viral damage due to cell cytolysis and an interruption of mitosis, or from endothelial injury to the blood vessels affecting the cochlear duct, vascular stricture, or alteration in endolymph levels. The characteristics of hearing loss usually include the following features:

- Neurosensory type
- Often of profound grade

- Bilateral involvement
- Symmetrical
- Irreversible
- It may have late presentation.

Immunization with effective vaccines has practically eliminated the occurrence of congenital rubella. This confirms the importance of vaccination awareness programs.

3.1.6 Varicella zoster

The varicella-zoster virus initially causes chickenpox, and in case of reactivation, it becomes herpes zoster [12]. The auricular aspect of herpes zoster, called herpes zoster oticus, is characterized by otalgia – especially pain in the pinna and its vesicles, usually in the concha or external auditory meatus, and in the oral mucosa [23].

Ramsay Hunt Syndrome is diagnosed when, along with the condition described above, unilateral facial paralysis occurs. The syndrome is rare, with less than 1% of cases of varicella zoster infection resulting in the syndrome. It is more prevalent in the elderly (between the 6th and 7th decades of life) and rare in children [24].

The varicella-zoster virus remains in the spinal and cranial ganglia after the first infection (chickenpox). Numerous conditions can reactivate the virus and cause its replication, among them:

- Individuals not immunized against chickenpox
- Immunosuppressed individuals
- Newborns
- Pregnant women
- Individuals under physical and/or emotional stress.

The use of antivirals and steroids effectively reduces late complications. The faster the response to treatment, the better the prognosis.

In a literature review of cochleovestibular disorders in Herpes Zoster Oticus, Teggi et al. (2023) [23] included 38 studies in which the findings were controversial. Cases of sensorineural hearing loss with descending configuration have been reported, i.e., hearing loss is more prevalent at high frequencies to a mild to moderate degree. In most studies, hearing loss showed cochlear or retrocochlear features. The hearing loss seems to result from inflammation of the geniculate ganglion of the VIII cranial nerve. In addition, alterations have been observed in vestibular examinations, showing dysfunction at the level of the semicircular canals; dysfunction has also been seen in the function of the otolytic organs, as revealed by alterations in myogenic evoked potentials (VEMPs). Most of the studies reviewed by Teggi et al. found that hearing loss was transient, as was tinnitus, so that at the end of a successful treatment, patients regained their hearing.

3.1.7 SARS-CoV-2 (COVID-19)

Coronavirus disease 2019 (COVID-19), caused by the SARS-CoV-2 virus [12], was initially reported in Wuhan, Hubei Province, China, and has spread globally, impacting more than 120 countries and becoming a global public health concern [25]. COVID-19 transmission occurs predominantly through the respiratory route, although research has shown the possibility of vertical transmission, in which the virus is transferred from mother to fetus (through either viral particles in the amniotic fluid, through the placenta, from exposure to contaminated maternal blood or secretions, or during breastfeeding) [26].

The mechanisms by which SARS-CoV-2 can cause hearing loss are multifaceted, as there are many strains of the virus. The virus can damage the auditory areas of the brain and the cochlea. The symptoms of the disease are:

- Fever or chills
- Cough
- Fatigue
- Muscle or body pain
- Headache
- Sore throat
- Congestion or runny nose
- Shortness of breath or difficulty breathing
- Recent loss of smell or taste.

In addition, there are other less common symptoms, such as nausea or vomiting, diarrhea, blisters or swelling in the fingers, and conjunctivitis.

Raimundo et al. (2024) conducted one of the first prospective, cross-sectional, and longitudinal studies where BAEPs (Brainstem Auditory Evoked Potentials) were used to diagnose hearing loss [27]. The researchers did not identify hearing loss in any of the infants evaluated, although some abnormal BAEP latencies were seen. Transient evoked otoacoustic emissions (TEOAEs) were also studied, and it was observed that there were reduced responses at higher frequencies, raising the possibility of damage to the hair cells in the basal spiral [27]. These findings corroborate the review of Mitsikas et al. (2021), who point to damage to cochlear structures in individuals exposed to pathogens in cases of fetal viral infections [28].

Siqueira et al. [29] investigated the audiological patterns of children and adolescents affected by SARS-CoV-2, finding hearing thresholds within normal limits for all participants [29]. However, they did identify a lack of responses at high frequencies in otoacoustic emissions and weaker acoustic reflexes, which indicate changes in hair cells and afferent and efferent pathways, perhaps caused by COVID-19. Supplementary tests to evaluate the central auditory system also showed altered responses in infected children and adolescents [29].

Regarding hearing alterations, there is little information on the effect of SARS-CoV-2, with most studies being retrospective and focusing on screening procedures (there are few prospective studies including diagnostic tests and few longitudinal studies). However, a meta-analysis published in 2022, which reviewed 26 studies, reported the effects of COVID-19 on the auditory and vestibular systems, identifying the presence of dizziness in 17.8%, tinnitus in 8.1%, and vertigo in 2.8% of cases [30]. Although there was variability in findings among the different studies, the following audiological features were found:

- Sensorineural or conductive type
- Variable degree
- Unilateral or bilateral involvement
- Symmetrical or asymmetrical
- Sudden or not
- There is no pattern

However, it is important to note that peripheral audiological evaluations still need to be conducted to determine whether COVID infection causes any permanent damage to the auditory system. The causal relationship between COVID and hearing loss still lacks scientific evidence from controlled clinical studies.

3.1.8 Measles

Measles is an acute, highly transmissible viral disease caused by an RNA virus of the genus *Morbillivirus* of the Paramyxoviridae family. The pathogen is a single-strand RNA virus that is easily transmitted either by contact with respiratory secretions or by vertical transmission (mother–fetus) [12, 31].

The symptoms of the disease are:

- Fever or chills
- Cough
- Nasal congestion
- Intense discomfort

- Eye irritation
- Maculopapular exanthem (red spots)
- Koplik spots on the oral mucosa (a pathognomic sign of measles).

Before the development of vaccines, measles was the causative agent of 5% to 10% of profound sensorineural hearing loss in the United States. In the year 2000, it was considered eradicated in the U.S., although cases resulting from immigration or importation of the virus are still reported. In countries where the vaccination rate or access to vaccines is low, measles remains one of the most frequent causes of profound hearing loss.

The measles virus has been implicated in congenital hearing loss secondary to intrauterine infection, in idiopathic sudden hearing loss in adults and children [32, 33], and in hearing loss acquired after natural measles infection [34]. Hearing loss due to intrauterine measles infection is usually severe and associated with multiple, apparently rare, and unrelated congenital anomalies. Measles may also be related to a greater propensity for otitis media due to decreased immunity during treatment.

The pathophysiology of hearing loss is associated with the degeneration of cochlear neurons in the basal gyrus of the cochlea, as well as the degeneration of the organ of Corti and the stria vascularis. Therefore, depending on the topodiagnosis, hearing loss can exhibit cochlear or retrocochlear characteristics. The characteristics of hearing loss usually follow the following pattern:

- Neurosensory type
- Moderate to profound grade
- Typically bilateral
- Irreversible.

The most effective treatment against hearing loss due to measles infection is vaccination, which is indicated for babies from 12 months. In the literature, there are some reports about vaccine-induced encephalitis that can also result in hearing loss [35, 36]. However, this association is still unclear and needs further study.

If hearing loss has occurred, treatment should be based on providing a suitable hearing device, which can vary from hearing aids and/or cochlear implants, depending on the type and degree of hearing impairment.

3.1.9 Mumps

Mumps is a highly contagious disease caused by the same family of viruses as rubella and measles [12]. The pathogen responsible is the mumps virus, a member of the Paramyxoviridae family, usually of the genus *Paramyxovirus*. It is transmitted, predominantly horizontally, by respiratory secretions and is one of the most common causes of acquired unilateral sensorineural hearing loss of sudden onset [37]. Its incidence is extremely variable between studies, probably due to different vaccination practices among nations. Symptoms of mumps include:

- Fatigue
- Weakness
- Loss of appetite and pain when chewing and swallowing
- Pain and swelling in the salivary glands
- Swelling of the bilateral parotid glands
- Pancreatitis
- Orchitis (inflammation of the testicles)
- Oophoritis (inflammation of the ovaries)
- Infertility
- Flu-like symptoms.

Histological studies of temporal bones have shown results similar to those of individuals affected by measles and rubella, demonstrating that hearing loss occurs due to degeneration of the hair cells of the organ of Corti and the stria vascularis, in addition to damage to the myelin sheath around the VIII cranial nerve [31, 37]. The characteristics of hearing loss are:

- Neurosensory type
- Unilateral
- Severe to profound degree
- Tinnitus can coexist
- Vertigo can coexist
- Sudden.

There is no treatment for mumps except vaccination, which was introduced in 1949 and has drastically reduced its incidence. The vaccination schedule includes three doses: between 12 and 15 months, between 4 and 6 years of age, and at the end of adolescence. Examination of cases of mumps has revealed that their carriers had an incomplete vaccination schedule, indicating that campaigns for complete vaccination are still necessary.

3.2 Auditory manifestations of specific bacterial infections

Bacterial infections can cause a variety of auditory manifestations, some of which are acute and potentially reversible, while others can lead to permanent damage and long-term sequelae.

3.2.1 Bacterial meningitis

Bacterial meningitis is recognized as a leading cause of acquired deafness, with approximately 8% of survivors experiencing some degree of permanent hearing loss [38]. The pathogenic agents are several bacteria, the most common being *Streptococcus pneumoniae* and *Neusseria meningitidis* [12].

The symptoms of the disease are:

- High fever
- Vomiting
- Dis-ease
- Severe headache
- Stiff neck
- Red spots
- Alterations of consciousness
- Seizures
- Tinnitus

The pathology requires immediate treatment with antibiotics; vaccination is the best method of prevention. The exact mechanism of hearing loss in bacterial meningitis is not completely understood, but it is likely to involve multiple factors, such as the spread of infection to Corti's organ, ischemic damage with involvement of the peripheral and central auditory pathways, ossification of the cochlea, and increased endolymph levels leading to labyrinthitis [35, 36]. The hearing loss usually follows the following pattern:

- Neurosensory type
- Severe to profound degree
- Bilateral involvement
- Sudden
- Irreversible.

Hearing loss due to meningitis usually occurs around the second day of infection [39]. Thus, if proper treatment is carried out early, hearing loss can be reversed [40]. It is recommended that all children undergo a hearing test within 4 weeks of recovery from meningitis.

There is some controversy about the percentage of children with hearing loss as a result of meningitis. In a study by Kutz et al. [10], 30.6% of children diagnosed with meningitis had sensorineural hearing loss during audiological tests. In 41.4% of the cases, the hearing loss was mild or moderate, while in 58.6% of the cases, the hearing loss was severe or profound. Patients who developed hearing loss required longer hospitalization compared to those who maintained normal hearing [10].

A study by Persson et al. [41] examined the relationships between risk factors and hearing impairment in patients treated for bacterial meningitis in Sweden between 2000 and 2017 [41]. Of the 119 patients who had audiological test results in their medical records, 71 (59.6%) were diagnosed with some degree of hearing loss, with severe hearing loss being most frequent and usually involving the highest frequencies. The bacterium *Streptococcus pneumoniae* was present in 58% of cases. The coexistence of acute otitis media (AOM) was a risk factor associated with a negative outcome, with an odds ratio of 2.1:1. The authors suggest that otoscopy should be mandatory when patients are admitted with suspected bacterial meningitis, and if AOM is diagnosed, it should be treated with medications and myringotomy to reduce the risk of hearing loss [41].

3.2.2 Acute otitis media and chronic otitis media

Acute otitis media (AOM) is an infection in the auditory system caused by bacteria or viruses. The infection often originates from other illnesses, such as a cold, the flu, or an allergy.

AOM is very common and is one of the main reasons for medical care and the prescription of antibiotics [42]. Research in developed nations indicates that by about 3 years of age, 80% of children will have experienced at least one episode of the condition [43]. As with most infectious diseases, the incidence of AOM varies significantly between nations. The main disparities focus on the occurrence of suppurative complications, such as mastoiditis and meningitis, and the presence of sequelae, such as hearing loss resulting from chronic suppurative otitis media (COM) [42, 43]. Hearing loss due to COM is preventable and is a concern in developing countries, especially among children, since it can have lasting effects on early communication, language development, and auditory processing; it also affects psychosocial and cognitive development and educational performance.

Risk factors for the development of AOM include allergies, passive smoking, bottle-feeding, inadequate breastfeeding, upper respiratory tract infections, low socioeconomic status, previous history of AOM, adenoid hypertrophy, adenotonsillitis, day care attendance, low maternal educational attainment, and maternal smoking during pregnancy [44–46].

The main symptoms of AOM differ between children and adults.

Children:

- Earache

- Irritability and frequent crying
- Difficulty sleeping
- Fever
- Decreased appetite
- Discharge from the ear
- Hearing loss.

Adults:

- Earache
- Aural plenitude
- Hearing loss
- Discharge from the ear
- Tinnitus
- Dizziness
- Fever and general malaise.

Secretions filling the middle ear space surrounding the auditory ossicles (malleus, incus, and stapes) dampen vibration and hinder the transmission of sound to the inner ear. This results in a hearing loss that impairs low-pitched sounds, including speech. In the case of AOM, the loss may be temporary, and hearing returns to normal after treatment and fluid reabsorption. However, in cases of COM, where there has been chronic and repetitive inflammation, permanent damage to the tympanic membrane, ossicles, and the inner part of the inner ear can occur. Worsening of the condition can lead to the development of cholesteatoma, which is an abnormal growth of tissue that can expand to fill the external auditory canal and nearby areas. The characteristics of the hearing loss are:

- Conductive type
- Mild to moderate degree
- Usually bilateral, but can be unilateral
- In the case of COM, it can be reversed, but is irreversible if not properly addressed.

The early diagnosis and treatment of AOM, encompassing the rational use of antibiotics, are essential and will help prevent complications and long-term sequelae. The repercussions of otitis media for children can be serious, especially in terms of impairments to language development and school performance resulting from hearing loss [47–51]. Treatment of AOM can prevent the development of other pathologies, such as COM and cholesteatoma.

Health policies and programs for AOM and COM need to focus on preventive interventions, as well as improving access to effective care.

3.3 Antimicrobial drug-induced ototoxicity

Ototoxic drugs are those that have the potential to compromise the organs of balance and hearing. One pathophysiological mechanism is oxidative stress, which culminates in cell death. However, more studies are still needed to more clearly determine the pathophysiology of the effects of ototoxic drugs on the peripheral and central auditory systems [52].

Identifying and understanding ototoxic drugs is crucial in clinical practice, as these substances can have significant consequences for hearing. Common classes of ototoxic drugs include: platinum-based chemotherapeutic agents, aminoglycoside antibiotics, loop diuretics, salicylates (nonsteroidal anti-inflammatory drugs, NSAIDs), macrolide antibiotics, quinine, glycopeptide antibiotics (e.g., vancomycin), phosphodiesterase-5 (PDE5) inhibitors (e.g., sildenafil), and vinca alkaloids (e.g., vincristine) [52].

Aminoglycosides remain a cornerstone for treating life-threatening gram-negative infections worldwide. In many low- and middle-income settings, their low cost, room-temperature stability, and activity against resistant organisms often make them the only practical option for critically ill patients. The likelihood of aminoglycoside-related hearing damage increases with the total dose received and the length of therapy and is heightened by predisposing factors such as impaired renal function, advanced age (notably in neonates, whose distinct pharmacokinetics can drive excessively high drug levels), concomitant use of nephrotoxic agents, and specific mitochondrial variants that confer greater genetic susceptibility [9, 53].

Antimicrobial drugs can cause ototoxicity through accumulation in the hair cells of the inner ear. The buildup leads to the production of free radicals, which damage and eventually kill these cells. In addition, the production of free radicals leads to oxidative stress and damages hair cells. Other substances can also directly affect the structures of the inner ear, such as the stria vascularis, which is essential for cochlear function and for the production and absorption of endolymph [53, 54].

Antimicrobial therapy can preserve cochlear hair cells through strategies including the use of antioxidants, modulation of inflammatory signaling pathways, and pharmacokinetic adjustments that minimize inner-ear exposure. Identifying biomarkers of drug-related ototoxicity prior to treatment facilitates risk stratification, thereby informing which patients require enhanced monitoring and preventive interventions. Pre-treatment genetic screening is not currently standard practice; however, targeted testing in high-risk populations, such as patients with pulmonary tuberculosis requiring aminoglycosides or cancer patients undergoing cisplatin treatment, may facilitate individualized care by balancing therapeutic advantages with the risk of hearing loss [53, 55].

The implications of exposure to ototoxic factors can be diverse and vary from person to person. The characteristics of hearing loss usually involve:

- Neurosensory type
- Impairment especially in high frequencies
- Progressive loss can extend to mid and low frequencies
- Variable degree
- Sudden or gradual
- Transient or permanent
- Tinnitus
- Dizziness
- Vertigo
- Imbalance
- Aural plenitude.

A clinical diagnosis of ototoxicity depends on comparing two audiological examinations: one before and another after exposure to an ototoxic substance. Nevertheless, it is still rare for this procedure to be routinely done in most patients – i.e., the lack of an audiological test before treatment with an ototoxic drug begins is a major obstacle to identifying hearing loss. Often, the administration of an ototoxic drug is an emergency response, as in the case of aminoglycosides, effectively ruling out an audiological test before treatment begins. In this situation, the presence of a multidisciplinary team is important in order to support these patients.

3.4 Functional decline of the immune system associated with aging

The functional decline of the immune system associated with aging significantly contributes to the increased susceptibility to infections in elderly adults, but paradoxically also results in inflammatory dysregulation affecting multiple organ systems, including the inner ear. With age, the distribution of lymphocyte subpopulations changes dramatically, resulting in impaired responsiveness to new pathogens. Production of pro-inflammatory cytokines by the aging immune system remains chronically elevated compared to the young, thus, auditory structures are damaged when present in sustained increased concentrations [56, 57].

3.5 Genetic therapy for hereditary and acquired hearing disorders

The treatment of hearing loss through gene therapy has advanced significantly, especially in cases of profound deafness associated with mutations in the OTOF gene. Initial clinical evidence indicated the restoration of auditory function in affected children. In this trial, 10 out of 11 participants who received the adenoviral vector containing a functional version of OTOF showed remarkable improvements, with some patients reaching nearly normal hearing levels. While initial research efforts focused on hereditary single-gene genetic disorders, the ongoing development of gene editing paves the way for treating acquired hearing problems, such as those resulting from ototoxins or infections, by correcting mutations in auditory cells. The biggest technical obstacle in gene therapy for the auditory system lies in the effective delivery of genetic material to the target cells in the cochlea. This challenge is exacerbated by the isolated nature of this organ, which has a blood-labyrinth barrier that restricts the access of large molecules, such as viral vectors. Recently, research has made significant progress with the identification of DNA regulatory elements that are specifically active in cochlear support cells. This knowledge has enabled the creation of adeno-associated virus vectors that activate the therapeutic gene load only in support cells, preventing activation in other cochlear cells and consequently reducing potential side effects. The future of auditory gene therapy points toward the combination of this approach with the use of neurotrophic factors and apoptosis inhibitors. This strategy aims to maximize the recovery of auditory function by optimizing the regeneration of hair cells from residual supporting cells, exploring the convergence of multiple signaling pathways for an enhanced functional outcome [58].

3.6 Inflammation in the pathogenesis of multiple types of hearing loss

Due to the increasingly recognized role of inflammation in the origin of various forms of acquired hearing loss, current research has focused on exploring anti-inflammatory interventions. The objective of these strategies is not only to preserve hearing after damage caused by infections or ototoxic medications but also to offer the possibility of restoring lost auditory function [59–61]. Systemic corticosteroids are widely used in the treatment of idiopathic sudden sensorineural hearing loss and other inflammatory conditions. Studies indicate that this approach can result in a clinically detectable improvement in about 30% to 65% of patients, with more favorable outcomes observed in younger individuals or those with initially milder hearing loss. As an alternative for patients who cannot receive systemic corticosteroids or as rescue therapy for those who do not respond to initial treatment, tympanic therapy offers a viable option. This technique involves the injection of dexamethasone directly into the middle ear space. Research suggests that this local administration provides an additional benefit when applied within the first two to six weeks after the onset of symptoms. Another promising area of research involves JNK inhibitors (c-Jun N-terminal kinase). JNK is a protein kinase that is activated in response to cellular stress and plays a role in mediating inflammation-induced apoptosis. In animal models, JNK inhibition has demonstrated the ability to reduce hearing loss caused by a variety of stressors, such as noise, ototoxins, and inflammation. Currently, several JNK inhibitor compounds are in preclinical development phases and early clinical trials for the treatment of hearing loss [53, 62–64].

4. Final thoughts

Hearing health is directly related to well-being and communication with peers. The processes that lead to hearing damage are diverse, ranging from direct damage to the structures of the inner ear caused by pathogens, as occurs in measles and meningitis, to inflammatory and immune-mediated reactions, such as in congenital toxoplasmosis and COVID-19.

Immunosuppression, such as that seen in HIV, makes the body more susceptible to secondary infections that can affect hearing. Also, the ototoxicity of antimicrobial drugs, including both aminoglycosides and some antiretroviral medications, constitutes a considerable iatrogenic risk.

The pathogenic complexity involved underlines the importance of diagnosis and management, including infectious disease specialists, audiologists, and neurologists. Because viral infections can cause a multiplicity of auditory manifestations – ranging from congenital hearing loss due to CMV, sensorineural hearing loss due to measles, mumps, and HIV, and new associations from SARS-CoV-2 – medicos need to be aware of all these possibilities so that a hearing test becomes an essential component of the diagnostic repertoire. Comprehensive and personalized audiological screening and long-term follow-up for affected children will promote full speech and language development.

Ototoxicity is a widespread risk and goes beyond aminoglycosides, encompassing antiretroviral treatments. There are multiple risk factors to hearing, including exposure to noise and co-infections. For vulnerable populations, constant audiological monitoring and referral to drug control guidelines are needed.

5. Recommendations

1. **Increasing immunization coverage:** Continued and planned support for immunization programs, particularly in low- and middle-income nations, to prevent hearing loss caused by infections such as measles, mumps, and bacterial meningitis.

2. **Scaling up hearing screening programs:** Implementing and reinforcing universal newborn audiological screening, along with targeted screening for children and adults at risk after specific infections (e.g., meningitis, congenital toxoplasmosis, COVID-19) or exposure to ototoxic medications; investing in hearing screening of schoolchildren to detect acquired hearing loss that may compromise learning.

3. **Coordination of multidisciplinary care:** Encourage multidisciplinary teams (audiologists, otolaryngologists, pediatricians, infectious disease specialists, nephrologists, and neurologists) to diagnose and manage complex auditory

manifestations, ensuring comprehensive evaluations and individualized treatment plans.

4. **Ototoxicity control:** Patients who have taken or are using ototoxic medications should be tested and monitored regularly, making it possible to intervene early and prevent loss.

5. **Awareness and education programs:** Dissemination of information on the auditory manifestations of infectious diseases to health professionals and the general population.

6. **Longitudinal surveys:** Longitudinal surveys provide important data on the benefits of drug and audiological interventions, as well as giving insights into areas for improvement, allowing new treatments and research directions to be explored.

6. Conclusions

Good understanding of the auditory manifestations of infectious diseases is a primary step in improving the prevention, diagnosis, and treatment of these conditions. The motivation is to preserve and/or rehabilitate hearing, thereby promoting the fullest development of every individual.

Author details

Milaine Dominici Sanfins[1,2,3]*, Daniela Gil[1,2] and Piotr Henryk Skarzynski[3,4]

1 Department of Speech-Hearing-Language, Universidade Federal de São Paulo, São Paulo, Brazil

2 Post-Graduate Program in Clinical Audiology, Albert Einstein Institute of Education and Research , São Paulo, Brazil

3 Department of Teleaudiology and Screening, World Hearing Center, Institute of Physiology and Pathology of Hearing, Warsaw, Poland

4 Department of Otolaryngology, Institute of Sensory Organs, Warsaw, Poland

*Address all correspondence to: msanfins@uol.com.br; msanfins@unifesp.br

References

[1] Van Seventer JM, Hochberg NS. Principles of infectious diseases: transmission, diagnosis, prevention, and control. In: Quah SR, Cockerham WC, editors. International Encyclopedia of Public Health. 2nd ed. San Diego (CA): Elsevier; 2017. p. 22–39

[2] Coyne CB, Lazear HM.Zika virus—reigniting the TORCH. Nature Reviews Microbiology. 2016;**14**(11):707–715

[3] Helmi N, Alammari D, Mobashir M. Role of potential COVID-19 immune system associated genes and the potential pathways linkage with Type-2 diabetes. Combinatorial Chemistry & High Throughput Screening. 2022;**25** (14):2452–2462

[4] Perelson AS, Rong L, Hayden FG. Combination antiviral therapy for Influenza: Predictions from modeling of human infections. The Journal of Infectious Diseases. 2012;**205**(11): 1642–1645

[5] Screaton G, Mongkolsapaya J, Yacoub S, Roberts C. New insights into the immunopathology and control of dengue virus infection. Nature Reviews Immunology. 2015;**15**(12):745–759

[6] Błaszkowska J, Góralska K. Clinical cases of parasitoses and fungal infections important from medical point of view. Annals of Parasitology. 2016;**62** (4):255–265

[7] Jones KE, Patel NG, Levy MA, Storeygard A, Balk D, Gittleman JL, et al. Global trends in emerging infectious diseases. Nature 2008;**451**:9903

[8] Johri M, Téhinian S, Pérez Osorio MC, Barış E, Wahl B. Vaccination for prevention of hearing loss: A scoping review. Communications Medicine. 2025;**5**(1):85

[9] Rivetti S, Romano A, Mastrangelo S, Attinà G, Maurizi P, Ruggiero A. Aminoglycosides-related ototoxicity: Mechanisms, risk factors, and prevention in pediatric patients. Pharmaceuticals (Basel). 2023;**16** (10):1353. DOI: 10.3390/ph16101353

[10] Kutz JW, Simon LM, Chennupati SK, Giannoni CM, Manolidis S. Clinical predictors for hearing loss in children with bacterial meningitis. Archives of Otolaryngology–Head & Neck Surgery. 2006;**132**(9):941–945

[11] Ramchandani MS, Litvack JR, Marra CM. Otosyphilis: A review of the literature. Sexually Transmitted Diseases. 2020;**47**(5):296–300

[12] Shi X, Liu X, Sun Y. The pathogenesis of cytomegalovirus and other viruses associated with hearing loss: Recent updates. Viruses. 2023;**15**(6):1385

[13] Aldè M, Binda S, Primache V, Pellegrinelli L, Pariani E, Pregliasco F, et al. Congenital cytomegalovirus and hearing loss: The state of the art. Journal of Clinical Medicine. 2023;**12**:4465

[14] Ferreira L, Sanfins MD, Pinto JD, Skarzynski PH, Skarynska MB, Biaggio EPV. Congenital toxoplasmosis and auditory disorders: A literature review. Frontiers in Psychology. 2024;**14**:1286211

[15] Capra D, Dos Santos MF, Sanz CK, Acosta Filha LG, Nunes P, Heringer M, et al. Pathophysiology and mechanisms

of hearing impairment related to neonatal infection diseases. Frontiers in Microbiology. 2023;**14**:1162554

[16] Matas CG, Angrisani RG, Magliaro FC, Segurado AA. Audiological manifestations in HIV-positive adults. Clinics (Sao Paulo). 2014;**69**:469–475

[17] Peter VZ, Paken J, Joseph L. An audiological profile of a cohort of school-aged children with HIV and AIDS attending an antiretroviral clinic in South Africa. South African Journal of Communication Disorders. 2020;**67**:0–9

[18] Lin C, SW L, Weng SF, Lin YS. Increased risk of sudden sensorineural hearing loss in patients with human immunodeficiency virus aged 18 to 35 years: A population-based cohort study. JAMA Otolaryngology–Head & Neck Surgery. 2013;**139**(3):251–255

[19] Charles M, Nsirimobu P. Hearing disorders among HIV positive children at the University of Port Harcourt Teaching Hospital, Port Harcourt, Nigeria. Journal of Scientific Research and Reports. 2020;**25**(5):1–9

[20] Ezike E, Steele R Pediatric Rubella [Internet]. Medscape; 2025. Available from: https://emedicine.medscape.com/article/968523-overview [Accessed: 2025-September-02]

[21] CDC. Manual for the surveillance of vaccine-preventable diseases [Internet]. CDC; 2025 Chapter 15: Congenital Rubella Syndrome. Available from: https://www.cdc.gov/surv-manual/php/table-of-contents/chapter-15-congenital-rubella-syndrome.html [Accessed: 2025-September-02]

[22] Kadek K, Darmadi S. Congenital rubella symptoms based on serological and viral RNA examination Indonesia. Journal of Clinical Pathology and Medical Laboratory. 2007;**13**(2):63–71

[23] Teggi R, Del Poggio A, Cangiano I, Nobile A, Gatti O, Bussi M. Cochleo-vestibular disorders in herpes zoster oticus: A literature review and a case of bilateral vestibular hypofunction in unilateral HZO. Journal of Clinical Medicine. 2023;**12**(19):6206

[24] Goswami Y, Gaurkar SS. Ramsay hunt syndrome: An introduction, signs and symptoms, and treatment. Cureus. 2023;**15**(1):e33688

[25] Sriwijitalai W, Wiwanitkit V. COVID-19 outbreak in international airport—Where the incidence case occurs? International Journal of Preventive Medicine. 2020;**11**:51

[26] Sankaran D, Nakra N, Cheema R, Blumberg D, Lakshminrusimha S. Perinatal SARS-CoV-2 Infection and Neonatal COVID-19: A 2021 Update. NeoReviews. 2021;**22**:284–295

[27] Raimundo JQ, Sanfins MD, Skarzynski PH, Skarzyńska MB, Colella-Santos MF. Assessment of the peripheral and central auditory system in infants whose mothers tested positive for COVID-19 during pregnancy. Children (Basel, Switzerland). 2024;**11**:1527

[28] Mitsikas D, Gabrani C, Giannakou K, Lamnisos D. Intrauterine exposure to Zika virus and hearing loss within the first few years of life: A systematic literature review. International Journal of Pediatric Otorhinolaryngology. 2021;**147**:110801

[29] Siqueira J, Sanfins MD, Skarzynski PH, Skarzynska MB, Colella-Santos MF. Evaluation of the peripheral and central auditory systems in children and adolescents before and after

COVID-19 Infection. Children (Basel, Switzerland). 2024;**11**:1454

[30] Maleki M, Maarefvand M, Nazeri AR, Akbarzadeh BAR, Borna A. Audio-vestibular profile of COVID-19; systematic review and meta-analysis. Iranian Journal of Otorhinolaryngology. 2022;**34**(123):145–155

[31] Cohen BE, Durstenfeld A, Roehm PC. Viral causes of hearing loss: A review for hearing health professionals. Trends in Hearing. 2014;**18**:2331216514541361

[32] Tieri L, Masi R, Marsella P, Pinelli V. Sudden deafness in children. International Journal of Pediatric Otorhinolaryngology. 1984;**7**:257–264

[33] Veltri RW, Wilson WR, Sprinkle PM, Rodman SM, Kavish DA. The implication of viruses in idiopathic sudden hearing loss: Primary infection or reactivation of latent viruses. Otolaryngology–Head and Neck Surgery. 1981;**89**:137–141

[34] Lindsay JR, Hemenway WG. Inner ear pathology due to measles. Annals of Otology, Rhinology & Laryngology. 1981;**89**:1137–1141

[35] Rosenhal U, Nylen O, Lindenberg J, Kankkunen A. Auditory function after Haemophilus influenza meningitis. Acta Oto-Laryngologica. 1978;**85**:243–247

[36] Dodge PR, Davis H, Feigin RD, Holmes SJ, Kaplan SL, Luces-Ramos E, et al. Prospective evaluation of hearing impairment as a sequela of acute bacterial meningitis. New England Journal of Medicine. 1984;**311**: 869–874

[37] Paparella MM, Schachern PA. Sensorineural hearing loss in children—nongenetic. In: Paparella MM, Schumrick DA, Gluckman JL, Meyerhoff WL, editors. Otolaryngology. 3rd ed. Philadelphia (PA): Saunders; 1991. p. 1571–1572

[38] Edmond K, Clark A, Korczak VS, Sanderson C, Griffiths UK, Rudan I. Global and regional risk of disabling sequelae from bacterial meningitis: A systematic review and meta-analysis. The Lancet Infectious Diseases. 2010;**10** (5):317–328

[39] Richardson MP, Reid A, Tarlow MJ, Rudd PT. Hearing loss during bacterial meningitis [correction in Arch Dis Child. 1997; 76:386]. Archives of Disease in Childhood. 1997;**76**:134–138

[40] Bhatt SM, Lauretano AC, Cabellos C, Masure S, Tuomanen E, Syrogiannopoulos GA, et al. Progression of hearing loss in experimental pneumococcal meningitis: Correlation with cerebrospinal fluid cytochemistry. Journal of Infectious Diseases. 1993;**167**:675–683

[41] Persson F, Bjar N, Hermansson A, Gisselsson-Solen M. Hearing loss after bacterial meningitis, a retrospective study. Acta Oto-Laryngologica. 2022;**142**(3-4):298–301

[42] Klein JO. The burden of otitis media. Vaccine. 2000;**19**(Suppl 1): S2–S8

[43] Vergison A, Dagan R, Arguedas A, Bonhoeffer J, Cohen R, Dhooge I, et al. Otitis media and its consequences: Beyond the earache. The Lancet Infectious Diseases. 2010;**10**:195–203

[44] Songu M, Islek A, Imre A, Aslan H, Aladag I, Pinar E, et al. Risk factors for otitis media with effusion in children

with adenoid hypertrophy. Acta Otorhinolaryngologica Italica. 2020;**40**:133–135

[45] Zhang Y, Xu M, Zhang J, Zeng L, Wang Y, Zheng QY. Risk factors for chronic and recurrent otitis media–a meta-analysis. Public Library of Science One. 2014;**9**(1):e86397

[46] Vickers NJ. Animal communication: When I'm calling you, will you answer too? Current Biology. 2017;**27**(14):R713–R715

[47] Sanfins MD, Bertazolli LF, Skarzynski PH, Skarzynska MB, Donadon C, Colella-Santos MF. Otoacoustic emissions in children with long-term middle ear disease. Life (Basel, Switzerland). 2020;**10**(11):287

[48] Sanfins MD, Donadon C, Borges LR, Skarzynski PH, and Colella-Santos MF. Long-term effects of unilateral and bilateral otitis media and myringotomy on long-latency verbal and non-verbal auditory-evoked potentials. International Archives of Otorhinolaryngology. 2020;**24**(4):413–22

[49] Colella-Santos MF, Donadon C, Sanfins MD, Borges LR. Otitis media: Long-term effect on central auditory nervous system. BioMed Research International. 2019;**2019**:8930904

[50] Sanfins MD, Borges LR, Donadon L, Hatzopoulos S, Skarzynski PH, Colella-Santos MF. Electrophysiological responses to speech stimuli in children with otitis media. Journal of Health Science. 2017;**7**(4):9–19

[51] Sanfins MD, Skarzynski PH, Media C-SMFO. Behavioral and electrophysiological tests and auditory rehabilitation. In: Hatzopoulos S, Ciorba A, Skarzynski PH, editors. The Human Auditory System—Basic Features and Updates on Audiological Diagnosis and Therapy. London (UK): IntechOpen; 2019

[52] Sanfins MD, Skarzynska MB, Skarzynski PH, Gil D. The clinical implication of ototoxicity on the auditory system (part I): Hearing loss in vulnerable groups. MEDINCUS. 2025;**30**. DOI: 10.5281/ZENODO.15933145

[53] Fu X, Wan P, Li P, Wang J, Guo S, Zhang Y, An Y, Ye C, Liu Z, Gao J, Yang J, Fan J, Chai R. Mechanism and prevention of ototoxicity induced by aminoglycosides. Frontiers in Cellular Neuroscience. 2021;**15**:692762. DOI: 10.3389/fncel.2021.692762

[54] Yansey A, Harris MS, Egbelakin A, Gilbert J, Pisoni DB, Renbarger J. Risk factors for cisplatin-associated ototoxicity in pediatric oncology patients. Pediatric Blood & Cancer. 2012;**59**(1):144–148. DOI: 10.1002/pbc.24138

[55] Consortium AB, Xiaolong F, Wang S, Yunhao W, Sun Y, Liu W, Xin X, Geng-Lin L, Liu K, Yuan W, Chen F, Wang H, Yang T, Liu Y, Zheng J, Shi H, Jing Q, Chen X, Suo L, Huang Y, Xinbo X, Tang X, Xiaojun L, Lei X, Gao X, Lisheng Y, Shu Y, Zhang W, Sun J, Yuan H, Gong S, Wenyan L, Xiulan M, Zha D, Gao J, Huawei L, Zuhong H, Liu G-H, Pei G, Kong W, Wang H, Chai R. A biomarker framework for auditory system aging: The Aging Biomarker Consortium consensus statement. Life Medicine. 2025;**4**(1): lnaf011. DOI: 10.1093/lifemedi/lnaf011

[56] Yang W, Zhao X, Chai R, Fan J. Progress on mechanisms of age-related

hearing loss. Frontiers in Neuroscience. 2023;**17**:1253574

[57] Guo J, Huang X, Dou L, Yan M, Shen T, Tang W, Li J. Aging and aging-related diseases: From molecular mechanisms to interventions and treatments. Signal Transduction and Targeted Therapy. 2022;7(1):391

[58] Mittal R, Nguyen D, Patel AP, Debs LH, Mittal J, Yan D, Eshraghi AA, TR VDW, Liu XZ. Recent advancements in the regeneration of auditory hair cells and hearing restoration. Frontiers in Molecular Neuroscience. 2017;**10**:236

[59] Li L, Chen D, Lin X, Luo J, Tan J, Li P. Understanding the role of inflammation in sensorineural hearing loss: Current goals and future prospects. Brain Science Reviews. 2023;**3**(4):e34

[60] Li G, Yang H, Zhang P, Guo Y, Yuan L, Xu S, Yuan Y, Xiong H, Yin H. Insights into the molecular underlying mechanisms and therapeutic potential of endoplasmic reticulum stress in sensorineural hearing loss. Frontiers in Molecular Neuroscience. 2024;**17**:1443401

[61] Öztan G, İşsever H, Kurt ÖK, Canbaz S, Oğuz F, İşsever T, Öztürk Ö. Determination of differential miRNA expression profile in people with noise-induced hearing loss. International Journal of Molecular Sciences. 2025;**26**(14):6623. DOI: 10.3390/ijms26146623

[62] Tyagi S, Singh R, Tyagi A, Jain A. Onset of sudden sensorineural hearing loss: An update. Cureus. 2024;**16**(3): e56306

[63] Chen WT, Lee JW, Yuan CH, Chen RF. Oral steroid treatment for idiopathic sudden sensorineural hearing loss. Saudi Medical Journal. 2015;**36**(3):291–296. DOI: 10.15537/smj.2015.3.9940

[64] Chandrasekhar SS, Tsai Do BS, Schwartz SR, Bontempo LJ, Faucett EA, Finestone SA, Hollingsworth DB, Kelley DM, Kmucha ST, Moonis G, Poling GL, Roberts JK, Stachler RJ, Zeitler DM, Corrigan MD, Nnacheta LC, Satterfield L. Clinical practice guideline: Sudden hearing loss (update). Otolaryngology–Head and Neck Surgery: Official Journal of the American Academy of Otolaryngology-Head and Neck Surgery. 2019;**161**(1_suppl):S1–S45. DOI: 10.1177/0194599819859885

Chapter 3

Perspective Chapter: Blind Anti-Oxidation and Excessive Anti-Oxidation are Harmful to Normal Cells of the Inner Ear

Liling Li, Dalian Ding and Peng Li

Abstract

Oxidative stress is a core pathological mechanism in sensorineural hearing loss. It involves excessive production of reactive oxygen species and an imbalance in the antioxidant defense system. This imbalance damages key cells, such as inner ear hair cells and spiral ganglion neurons. However, blind or excessive antioxidant intervention can disrupt intracellular redox homeostasis and may trigger free radical chain reactions. For example, the Fenton reaction catalyzes the generation of hydroxyl radicals. Antioxidants themselves can also transform into free radical intermediates. These processes can paradoxically worsen cellular damage, a phenomenon known as the "antioxidant paradox". Clinical meta-analyses and experimental studies have confirmed this risk. For instance, high doses of N-acetylcysteine or the SOD mimetic M40403 can induce cochlear cell apoptosis. Current techniques for detecting oxidative stress have limitations. There is a lack of specific biomarkers, and obtaining tissue samples from the inner ear is difficult. These limitations prevent precise antioxidant therapy. Future strategies must shift toward targeted modulation. Examples include using hydrogen to selectively neutralize toxic free radicals or using metal chelators to block the source of radical generation. Another direction is the design of multifunctional antioxidants. The goal is to restore the redox balance rather than indiscriminately scavenging all free radicals.

Keywords: antioxidant paradox, free radical chain reaction, fenton reaction, hydroxyl radical, inner ear diseases

1. Introduction

Hearing loss represents a major global sensory disorder. It is a key modifiable factor that impairs social function and quality of life, while also significantly increasing the risk of dementia [1, 2]. Among its various forms, acquired sensorineural hearing loss, such as age-related and noise-induced types, ranks as a leading cause of disability [3]. The inner ear is a sensory organ with high metabolic activity. Its hair cells and spiral ganglion neurons, rich in mitochondria, are highly sensitive to redox imbalance. Under physiological conditions, a dynamic balance is maintained between reactive oxygen species (ROS) and the endogenous antioxidant system, with ROS participating in essential signal transduction. A disruption of this balance, whether tilting toward oxidative stress causing cell damage or toward excessive antioxidation leading to functional impairment, can trigger hearing loss [4].

Oxidative stress serves as a core pathological mechanism for various forms of acquired sensorineural hearing loss [5]. Research shows that the function and survival of inner ear hair cells and spiral ganglion neurons critically depend on the integrity of the antioxidant defense system. Deficiencies in key enzymes, such as SOD1 or glutathione reductase, significantly increase the cochlea's susceptibility to oxidative damage [6–10]. Excess ROS can activate cell death pathways, including apoptosis, necroptosis, and ferroptosis. This process often forms a vicious cycle with inflammatory responses, leading to irreversible auditory impairment. It also constitutes a common pathogenic basis for hearing loss associated with hypoxia, Meniere's disease, and diabetic auditory neuropathy. The molecular mechanisms involve a complex signaling network encompassing mitochondrial dysfunction, downregulation of SOD2, activation of PARP1, and dysregulation of non-coding RNAs [11–23].

However, the safety and efficacy of interventions targeting oxidative stress, particularly direct antioxidant approaches, are not self-evident. A key scientific question arises: are all forms of antioxidant intervention beneficial for inner ear cells? In reality, blind or excessive antioxidant use can interfere with the normal physiological signaling functions of ROS. It may even induce "reductive stress." This condition can similarly disrupt the redox homeostasis of inner ear cells and poses a potential threat to the normal function of hair cells and spiral ganglia. The damage caused by this imbalance in antioxidation is as significant as oxidative stress itself, yet it has not received sufficient attention. To fully understand this risk, we must examine the core mechanism of oxidative damage: the free radical chain reaction. Particular focus is needed on the hydroxyl radical, a highly reactive species generated through reactions catalyzed by transition metal ions like iron and copper. This process is a critical step through which oxidative stress causes widespread cellular damage. It also forms the molecular basis determining whether an antioxidant strategy will work and what potential side effects it may carry.

2. Free radical chain reactions and metal ion-mediated hydroxyl radical generation

Free radicals are highly reactive molecules containing unpaired electrons. They are widespread in biological systems and can be generated through endogenous metabolic processes. These processes include mitochondrial electron transport, enzymatic reactions, and the respiratory burst in immune cells. External factors, such as radiation, chemical toxins, and environmental pollutants, can also induce their production [24]. Under physiological conditions, free radicals act as crucial signaling molecules. They participate in cell proliferation, differentiation, apoptosis, and immune regulation. However, when free radical production exceeds the body's antioxidant defense capacity, oxidative stress occurs. This leads to oxidative damage of biological macromolecules like DNA, proteins, and lipids. Consequently, it contributes to the pathogenesis of various diseases, including neurodegenerative disorders, cardiovascular diseases, and tumorigenesis [24, 25].

Among the various reactive oxygen species, the hydroxyl radical possesses the highest reactivity. It has an extremely short half-life, approximately one nanosecond.

It can non-selectively attack nearly all biological molecules, causing severe oxidative damage [25]. The generation of hydroxyl radicals primarily relies on metal ion-catalyzed reactions. The Fenton reaction and Fenton-like reactions are central to this process. The core of these reactions involves transition metal ions, such as ferrous iron or cuprous copper, catalyzing the homolytic cleavage of hydrogen peroxide to yield the hydroxyl radical:

$$Fe^{2+} + H_2O_2 \rightarrow Fe^{3+} + \cdot OH + OH^-$$
$$Cu^{+} + H_2O_2 \rightarrow Cu^{2+} + \cdot OH + OH^-$$

It is noteworthy that the traditional view considered the Fenton reaction inefficient under physiologically neutral pH conditions. However, recent studies confirm that, in the presence of physiological ligands such as histidine, phosphate, or ATP, iron and copper can form soluble and highly reactive complexes. These complexes effectively catalyze the generation of hydroxyl radicals [25, 26]. For example, Wang and colleagues discovered that an iron-histidine complex can efficiently produce hydroxyl radicals via a Fenton-like reaction at neutral pH. Their work indicated that this pathway predominantly generates hydroxyl radicals rather than forming a high-valent iron-oxo species. This finding provides a new mechanism for understanding iron-mediated oxidative damage in neurodegenerative diseases [26].

Beyond iron, copper ions are also highly efficient catalysts for Fenton-like reactions. Research by Keshtkar Vanashi and others demonstrated that copper ions can catalyze hydroxyl radical production over a broader pH range, including physiological conditions, compared to iron systems. Their catalytic efficiency is modulated by their specific coordination environment [27]. Furthermore, certain pharmaceuticals, such as doxorubicin, can significantly enhance reactive oxygen species generation in the presence of metal ions. This effect is particularly pronounced under light exposure. These findings underscore the central catalytic role of metal ions in free radical chain reactions [28].

The damaging nature of free radicals lies in their chain reaction. An initial radical, such as superoxide anion, is converted to hydrogen peroxide by the enzyme superoxide dismutase. Hydrogen peroxide can then be transformed into the hydroxyl radical through metal ion catalysis. The hydroxyl radical rapidly attacks polyunsaturated fatty acids. This attack initiates a lipid peroxidation chain reaction. This process generates lipid radicals and lipid peroxyl radicals. These new radicals can then attack adjacent lipid molecules, thereby amplifying the damage [29]. A similar propagation occurs with proteins. An attack by a hydroxyl radical can generate a protein-based radical. This radical can then propagate oxidative damage to other molecules. This leads to protein cross-linking, aggregation, and ultimately, loss of function [30, 31]. When hydroxyl radicals attack DNA, they produce various oxidative adducts. One well-known example is 8-OHdG. This damage not only causes mutation accumulation, but studies using cochlear organoid models have confirmed that such oxidative damage can lead to neural axon degeneration. Supplementing with nicotinamide adenine dinucleotide was shown to be protective. This protection works by alleviating caspase-3-mediated apoptosis [32].

Crucially, antioxidant therapy itself can worsen this chain reaction if applied incorrectly. For instance, the SOD mimetic M40403 efficiently scavenges superoxide anion; however, this action can lead to an accumulation of hydrogen peroxide. If the cell's hydrogen peroxide clearance systems are inadequate, or if free metal ions are present, this excess hydrogen peroxide may be converted into the more toxic hydroxyl radical via the Fenton reaction [33, 34]. Similarly, antioxidants like N-acetylcysteine can auto-oxidize or interact with metal ions at high concentrations. This interaction can paradoxically promote the generation of hydroxyl radicals [35]. This mechanism explains findings from studies by Ding et al. and Li et al., where high concentrations of M40403, coenzyme Q10, and NAC actually increased apoptosis in cochlear hair cells and spiral neurons. Indiscriminate antioxidant intervention can disrupt the intracellular redox balance and may unintentionally activate metal-mediated free radical generation pathways, ultimately leading to damage in inner ear cells.

In summary, free radical damage is a chain reaction process that is catalyzed by metal ions and undergoes progressive amplification. Understanding this process does more than just reveal the molecular nature of oxidative stress; it also serves as a critical warning. Antioxidant therapies must be based on a precise assessment of the redox status. The goal is to avoid disrupting the endogenous balance and to prevent a well-intentioned "detoxification" from turning into a harmful "intoxication." However, significant limitations exist in our current technologies for detecting oxidative stress. These limitations directly hinder the precise application of antioxidant treatments. This is the key problem we will address next.

3. Limitations in oxidative stress detection and the non-specific use of antioxidants in inner ear disease

Although oxidative stress is recognized as a core pathological mechanism in many inner ear diseases, accurately assessing the redox state within the inner ear remains a major challenge in clinical practice. This is particularly true for localized assessment in hair cells and spiral ganglion neurons. This diagnostic gap directly leads to an empirical and non-specific approach to antioxidant therapy. Current methods for detecting free radicals and antioxidant enzymes are varied and can be broadly categorized.

Chemical and spectroscopic methods represent traditional mainstream techniques. These approaches indirectly evaluate oxidative stress levels through specific chemical reactions. Examples include using chemiluminescence assays to measure total antioxidant capacity or using free radical scavenging tests with compounds like ABTS cation radical or DPPH to assess a sample's antioxidant activity [30]. Fluorescent probe technology utilizes molecules that are selective for specific reactive oxygen species, such as hydrogen peroxide or the hydroxyl radical. This allows for real-time monitoring and imaging of intracellular ROS levels [4]. Furthermore, chromatography coupled with mass spectrometry techniques, including HPLC, LC–MS/MS, and GC–MS, can precisely separate and quantify specific antioxidant molecules or their oxidative modification products in biological samples. Measuring molecules like vitamin E, glutathione, or markers like 8-OHdG and MDA provides molecular evidence of oxidative damage [36].

Electrochemical methods have attracted significant interest due to their high sensitivity, rapid response, and potential for miniaturization. These techniques utilize electrodes modified with functional micro or nanomaterials, such as carbon nanotubes or metal nanoparticles. They employ methods like cyclic voltammetry or differential pulse voltammetry, allowing for the direct detection of redox-active substances, including hydrogen peroxide or superoxide anion, either in solution or on cell surfaces. They can also measure antioxidant concentrations. This capability offers the potential for real-time and in-situ monitoring [37–39].

Emerging technologies continue to advance the field. Nanozyme-based sensing is one such development. It uses certain nanomaterials, for instance, cerium oxide nanoparticles, to mimic the enzymatic activity of SOD or catalase. This enables the construction of sensors that are low-cost and highly stable, used for assessing antioxidant capacity [40]. More cutting-edge explorations involve quantum sensing technology. This approach is based on diamond nitrogen-vacancy centers. In theory, it allows for non-invasive, highly sensitive optical detection of free radicals at the single-cell level, even within tissue sections. This technology brings a revolutionary prospect for understanding free radical dynamics in pathological states. However, its application is currently still confined to basic research [41].

Despite the proliferation of techniques, these methods face fundamental limitations when applied to clinically diagnose oxidative stress within a specific organ or tissue.

A major challenge is the lack of standardization and specific biomarkers. There is currently no universally accepted "gold standard" biomarker that can comprehensively and accurately reflect the systemic or local oxidative stress status. Different detection methods assess different aspects, such as antioxidant potential, oxidative damage products, or specific ROS types. This leads to varied results that are difficult to compare directly. Consequently, clinical interpretation becomes challenging [41, 42].

A significant disconnect exists between in vitro assessment and the complex in vivo environment. Most high-throughput evaluations of antioxidant activity are performed in simplified laboratory systems. However, antioxidation within a living organism is a dynamic network. It is profoundly influenced by absorption, distribution, metabolism, transformation, and crosstalk among various cellular pathways. A substance demonstrating powerful antioxidant capacity in a test tube may fail inside the body. This failure can be due to low bioavailability, an inability to reach the site of pathology, or unexpected conversion into a pro-oxidant state. It might even become toxic [42–44]. Research on Alzheimer's disease provides a clear example. There, antioxidants often struggle to cross the blood-brain barrier and distribute effectively within neurons [44].

The intrinsic physicochemical properties of free radicals also present a major detection challenge. Free radicals, particularly the hydroxyl radical, have an extremely short lifespan, exceptionally high reactivity, and a very low steady-state concentration. These characteristics make their direct, quantitative, and in-situ detection exceptionally difficult. Current routine clinical tests, which measure markers like MDA or 8-OHdG in blood or urine, can only provide systemic, indirect, and delayed information about oxidative stress. They cannot precisely reflect the real-time redox status of a specific organ at a specific moment [4, 41].

A major diagnostic blind spot arises from the impracticality of tissue sampling. For organs like the inner ear, which is deeply embedded within the temporal bone and has a delicate, vital structure, obtaining living tissue for direct biochemical analysis is nearly impossible in clinical practice [4, 45]. Even emerging technologies like quantum sensing, which might work on ex vivo liver slices, cannot solve the challenge of achieving real-time, non-invasive, in vivo diagnosis for the inner ear.

These diagnostic limitations directly create a non-specific approach to clinical antioxidant therapy. When the presence and specific characteristics of oxidative stress in the inner ear remain unknown, any intervention based on "assumption" is essentially a shot in the dark. This lack of precision manifests in two key ways. First, the target of treatment is unclear. It is impossible to determine if hearing loss is primarily driven by active oxidative stress. This can lead to ineffective or even harmful interventions for patients who are not suitable candidates. Therefore, widely applying antioxidant therapy without precise diagnostics constitutes a form of hypothesis-based medical practice. It carries inherent iatrogenic risk and contradicts the "do no harm" principle. This is precisely why a deeper investigation is needed. Understanding how improper antioxidant intervention can disrupt or even amplify free radical chain reactions, ultimately damaging key auditory cells, is central to evaluating its risks. The following section will detail the potential harms of non-specific antioxidant treatment, from disturbing free radical kinetics to causing direct cell toxicity.

4. Potential harms of non-specific antioxidant therapy: From free radical chain reactions to cellular damage

The intracellular redox state is a precisely regulated, dynamic balancing system. Under physiological conditions, free radicals are produced through endogenous processes like mitochondrial respiration. They participate in critical functions such as cell signaling. Their levels are finely controlled by an endogenous antioxidant network that includes superoxide dismutase and glutathione [46–48]. However, excessive intervention with exogenous antioxidants can disrupt this delicate balance.

Research shows that exogenous antioxidants can rapidly intervene and modulate an oxidative-antioxidant imbalance. For instance, a 2024 randomized clinical trial demonstrated that healthy individuals, when subjected to an intense exercise challenge, showed a significant increase in red blood cell SOD activity after a single dose of superoxide dismutase derived from Bacillus amyloliquefaciens GF424. The treatment also activated glutathione peroxidase and lowered reactive oxygen species levels. Long-term supplementation sustainably elevated catalytic enzyme activities and increased reduced glutathione levels. It maintained redox balance by promoting the glutathione redox cycle and upregulating genes related to NADPH synthesis [49]. While this result highlights the regulatory potential of exogenous antioxidants, it more profoundly reveals the highly dynamic nature of the intracellular redox state. It implies that any external intervention must be applied with extreme caution to avoid interfering with the autonomous regulatory functions of this dynamic network.

The fundamental nature of free radical reactions is a chain process. The introduction of a single antioxidant often fails to stop the reaction; instead, it may catalyze the generation of more toxic free radical intermediates. For example, the SOD mimetic M40403 efficiently scavenges superoxide anion; however, this action simultaneously leads to an accumulation of hydrogen peroxide. If the cell's hydrogen peroxide clearance systems are insufficient, or if free transition metal ions are present, this hydrogen peroxide can be converted into the highly reactive hydroxyl radical via the Fenton reaction, paradoxically exacerbating oxidative damage [49, 50]. Indeed, research shows the protective effects of M40403 on the cochlea are context-dependent. It can protect hair cells from damage induced by gentamicin and paraquat, yet it offers no protection against the ototoxicity of cisplatin. This suggests that different causes of hearing loss may require distinct antioxidant strategies [51, 52]. Similarly, high concentrations of N-acetylcysteine can undergo auto-oxidation or interact with metal ions, and this interaction may unexpectedly promote the generation of hydroxyl radicals [53, 54]. Furthermore, salicylates, the active component of aspirin, can selectively induce spiral ganglion neuron death. They achieve this through a paradoxical upregulation of superoxide production, revealing a unique, oxidative stress-mediated neurotoxicity mechanism [55].

Our previous studies provide direct evidence for these mechanisms (**Figures 1–3**). Ding et al. found that treating cochlear explants with 50 μM M40403, coenzyme Q10, or D-methionine for 48 hours resulted in significant hair cell loss and damage to auditory nerve fibers [33]. Li et al. further confirmed that a high concentration of NAC reduced HEI-OC1 cell density by 30% to 50%, significantly lowered cell viability, and increased the proportion of apoptotic cells by four to five times. High concentrations of M40403 and coenzyme Q10 also caused a dose-dependent loss of cochlear hair cells and activated the caspase-3 apoptosis pathway [34]. These findings align with earlier research indicating that excessive use of a single antioxidant can disrupt the redox balance in inner ear cells, inducing a state of excessive antioxidation. It is important to note that the effects vary among different antioxidants. For instance, dietary vitamin C supplementation attenuated noise-induced hearing loss in a guinea pig model. In contrast, a deficiency in isocitrate dehydrogenase 2 accelerated age-related hearing loss in male mice by altering the cellular redox state [56, 57]. Furthermore, the efficacy of intervention is not guaranteed. In mice with a glutathione reductase deficiency, long-term, high-dose NAC treatment failed to effectively prevent age-related hearing loss and the progressive loss of inner hair cells [58]. Collectively, these studies demonstrate that the outcome of antioxidant intervention is highly dependent on the specific molecular target, the metabolic pathways involved, and the body's underlying redox status.

It is important to note that the effects of antioxidants are highly context-dependent. In vitro studies demonstrate that their outcomes rely on concentration, the specific microenvironment, and interactions with other molecules [59–61]. For instance, while vitamin E can protect model cell membranes from hydrogen peroxide-induced lipid oxidation [60], its indiscriminate supplementation may suppress physiological ROS signaling and disrupt normal cellular function [62].

In summary, the intracellular redox state is a dynamic and constantly shifting balance. Attempting to use a single antioxidant to "catalyze" or "scavenge" a specific free radical often fails to terminate the harmful chain reaction. Instead, it disrupts the body's precise antioxidant network. This disruption can generate more toxic secondary free radicals, ultimately leading to cell damage. Our preliminary experimental studies have confirmed that excessive use of single antioxidants, such as M40403, NAC, and coenzyme Q10, produces significant toxicity in normal cochlear cells. This harm is not an isolated laboratory finding. Numerous clinical meta-analyses also highlight the widespread risks associated with non-specific antioxidant therapy. The underlying molecular mechanisms of this "antioxidant paradox" require systematic elucidation.

5. Hazards of non-specific antioxidant therapy: From meta-analysis evidence to the "antioxidant paradox" molecular mechanism

A substantial body of clinical research and meta-analyses consistently shows that blind, excessive antioxidant therapy is often ineffective and may even increase

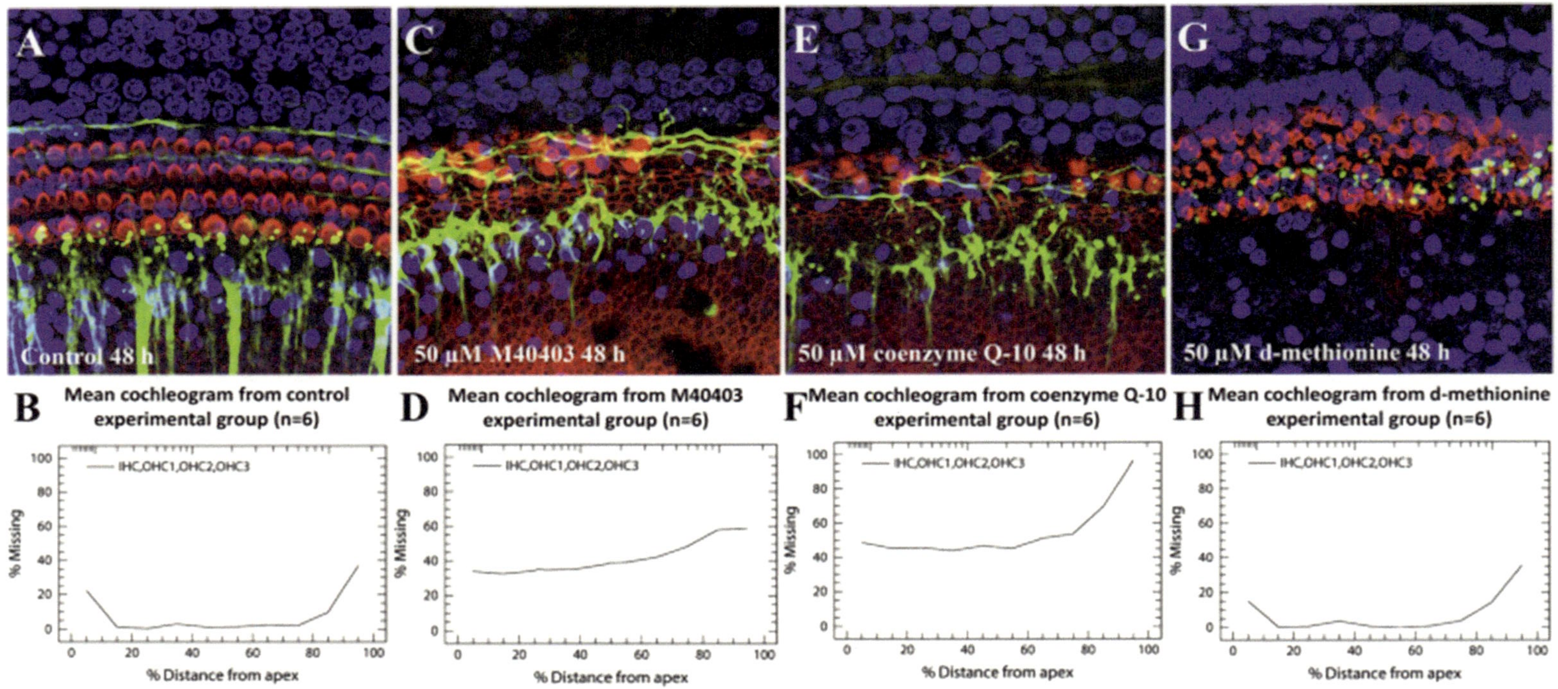

Figure 1.
High concentrations of antioxidants cause extensive hair-cell loss in cochlear explants. Representative images of the cochlear basilar membrane whole mount. Hair cell actin cytoskeleton is shown in red, stained with phalloidin. Auditory nerve terminals are shown in green, immunolabeled for beta-tubulin. Cell nuclei are shown in blue. Panels A and B show the control group after 48 hours in culture. Hair cells and nerve fibers exhibit normal morphology. Panels C and D show tissue treated with 50 µM M40403. This treatment leads to widespread hair cell loss. Panels E and F show tissue treated with 50 µM Coenzyme Q10. This treatment results in severe hair cell loss. Panels G and H show tissue treated with 50 µM D-methionine. This treatment also causes severe hair cell loss. The results demonstrate that high doses of M40403, Coenzyme Q10, and D-methionine induce significant hair cell loss along the entire length of the basilar membrane (Reproduced with permission from Ding et al, 2020).

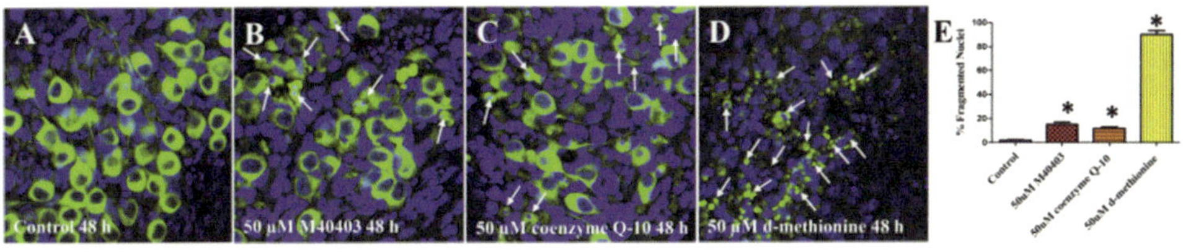

Figure 2.
High-dose antioxidant treatment induces degeneration of spiral ganglion neurons. Representative images of the spiral ganglion region are shown. Neuronal cell bodies are labeled in green using beta-tubulin immunofluorescence, while cell nuclei are stained blue. Panel A shows the control group, where neurons display normal morphology. Panel B shows tissue treated with M40403; this treatment leads to nuclear pyknosis in some neurons, as indicated by white arrows. Panel C shows tissue treated with Coenzyme Q10; this treatment triggers neuronal shrinkage with nuclear condensation, as indicated by white arrows. Panel D shows tissue treated with D-methionine; this treatment causes severe somatic shrinkage and nuclear fragmentation, as indicated by white arrows. Panel E presents quantitative statistics on the percentage of degenerated neurons. Data are shown as mean ± SEM, and an asterisk denotes a statistically significant difference compared to the control group (Reproduced with permission from Ding et al, 2020).

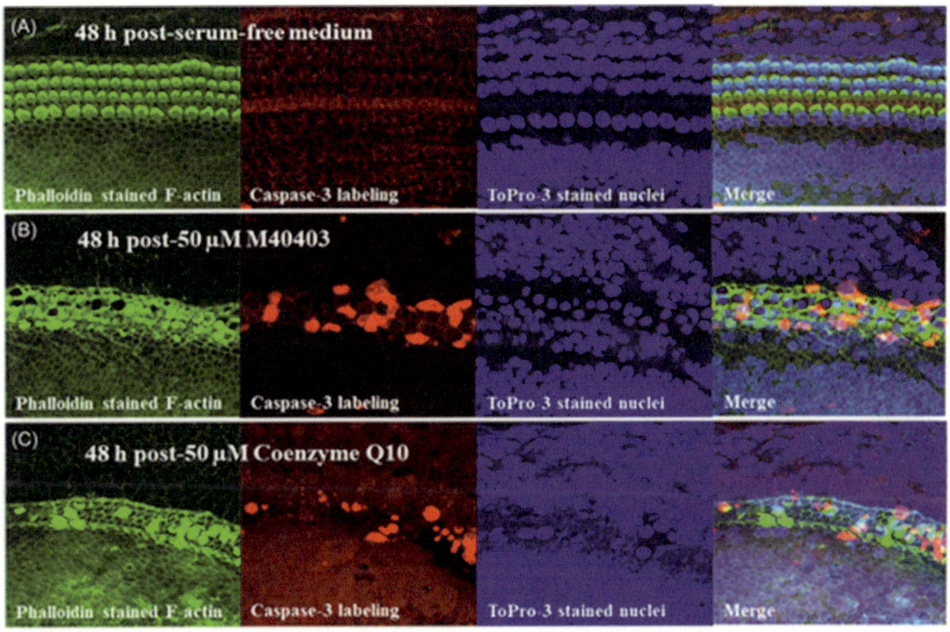

Figure 3.
High-concentration antioxidants induce cell death by activating the caspase-3 apoptosis pathway. The caspase-3 enzyme activity was significantly higher in treatment groups receiving high concentrations of antioxidants compared to the control group. This result indicates activation of the apoptotic pathway (Reproduced with permission from Li et al, 2024).

disease risk and mortality. A systematic review by Bjelakovic et al. focused on gastrointestinal cancer prevention and all-cause mortality. It found that various antioxidants, including beta-carotene, vitamin A, and vitamin E, showed no significant difference between intervention and control groups. Some antioxidants even potentially increased the incidence and mortality of certain cancers [63, 64].

Villanueva and Kross summarized antioxidant clinical trials from the past 15 years, involving 749,000 patients. They found that the number of cases not supporting the effectiveness of antioxidant therapy was 2.85 times greater than the number supporting its effectiveness. This strongly suggests the general ineffectiveness and potential harm of traditional single-agent antioxidant therapy in the overall population [65]. The deep-seated mechanism for this "ineffective or even harmful" phenomenon can be attributed to the "antioxidant paradox" triggered by non-specific antioxidant use. The concept was first formally proposed by Dündar and Aslan in 2000. It describes the redox homeostasis imbalance and resulting harm caused by an excess of exogenous antioxidants [66, 67]. When exogenous antioxidants are introduced in excessive amounts without precise diagnosis, particularly to cells or tissues not under severe oxidative stress, they disrupt the intrinsic intracellular redox homeostasis. This disruption triggers a chain of events that can ultimately lead to consequences more severe than the original oxidative damage. The core pathogenic mechanism lies in the unstoppable nature of free radical chain reactions and the "identity switch" characteristic of antioxidants. A free radical reaction is a dynamic, multi-step chain process. A specific antioxidant, like the SOD mimetic M40403, can efficiently scavenge its target radical. However, this action generates a downstream product. If the cell's subsequent clearance systems are inadequate, or if transition metal ions are present, this hydrogen peroxide can be converted into the more toxic hydroxyl radical via the Fenton reaction. In this scenario, an intervention intended to "detoxify" instead becomes a "generator" of more destructive radicals. More critically, an antioxidant itself, in the process of neutralizing a free radical, gains or loses an unpaired electron. It thereby transforms into a new free radical intermediate [68]. This newly formed radical, though potentially less active, can continue to participate in the chain reaction if not promptly cleared by downstream antioxidant systems. It may also transfer electrons to other biomolecules, expanding the scope of oxidative damage. For instance, high concentrations of N-acetylcysteine elevate glutathione levels. Yet, NAC or its metabolites can, under certain conditions, auto-oxidize or interact with metal ions. This interaction can paradoxically promote the generation of hydroxyl radicals [25].

Therefore, a higher dosage of an antioxidant is more likely to exceed the buffering capacity of the endogenous antioxidant network. This leads to the accumulation of more harmful free radical intermediates, creating a vicious cycle where the "antioxidant transforms into a free radical." This mechanism perfectly explains the experimental findings of Ding et al. and Li et al., where high concentrations of M40403, coenzyme Q10, and NAC directly induced caspase-3-mediated apoptosis in cochlear hair cells and spiral neurons. The excessive exogenous antioxidants disrupted the cell's precise redox regulation, ultimately triggering cell death through the "antioxidant paradox" mechanism [67]. Consequently, the damage caused by non-specific antioxidant use ultimately converges on the same pathway: oxidative damage to auditory functional cells. By catalyzing or participating in free radical chain reactions, they generate more toxic reactive oxygen species, such as the hydroxyl radical. This leads to a cascade of classic oxidative damage events, including lipid peroxidation, protein oxidation, and DNA damage. This means that a "one-size-fits-all" treatment approach, which ignores the local oxidative stress status in the inner ear, disregards dosage, and fails to consider the overall network balance, cannot protect the inner ear. Instead, it may act as an "accelerator" of cellular damage [69].

Antioxidant therapy is not a case of "more is better." Future progress must move beyond the traditional model of blindly supplementing single antioxidants. It must shift toward interventions designed to precisely restore redox homeostasis within the inner ear. Only this shift can truly circumvent the risk of "antioxidation" turning into "pro-oxidation," thereby providing a safe and effective path for hearing protection. Next, we will explore several novel antioxidant strategies that hold promise for achieving this goal.

6. Novel antioxidant strategies: From selective neutralization to source interdiction

Given the potential harm of indiscriminate antioxidant use to inner ear hair cells and spiral ganglion neurons, developing new strategies capable of precise intervention without disrupting normal redox homeostasis is crucial. The ideal approach should focus on two key directions: the first is the selective neutralization of the most toxic free radicals, and the second is the blockade of their generation at the source. This dual focus aims to protect auditory cells while preserving their physiological function.

6.1 Selective neutralization: The potential and limitations of hydrogen therapy

Hydrogen gas possesses a core advantage as a novel antioxidant. It selectively neutralizes highly toxic free radicals like the hydroxyl radical and peroxynitrite. In contrast, it has minimal effect on reactive oxygen species (ROS) with important signaling functions, such as hydrogen peroxide and superoxide anion [70, 71]. This property theoretically allows it to avoid disrupting normal physiological redox signaling in the inner ear, thereby circumventing the risk of the antioxidant paradox.

New material technologies are being employed to overcome the physical limitations of hydrogen gas, namely its low solubility and challenging administration. Research shows that hydrogen-rich water containing nano-sized bubbles can scavenge reactive oxygen species more efficiently. The mechanism may involve both direct ROS clearance and an indirect boost in the activity of endogenous antioxidant enzymes like glutathione peroxidase [72, 73]. A 2022 study combined nano-bubble technology with hydrogen water for the first time. It found that hydrogen nano-bubble water was highly effective at removing hydrogen peroxide and superoxide anion, significantly outperforming ordinarily dissolved hydrogen. The underlying mechanism may involve both direct scavenging and enhancing endogenous enzyme activity [74]. Furthermore, silicon-based agents are considered a breakthrough technology. They are thought to generate large amounts of antioxidative hydrogen in situ within the body. This action alleviates oxidative stress and also provides anti-inflammatory and anti-apoptotic effects [75]. This approach offers the potential for targeted delivery.

Although these technologies show promise in fields like cardiology and neurology, their application in inner ear diseases remains exploratory. A key question for future validation is whether they can effectively target and protect hair cells and spiral ganglia.

6.2 Source blocking: Metal ion chelation and multifunctional targeting strategies

An alternative root-cause approach focuses on blocking the generation of free radicals at their source rather than scavenging them after they form. The Fenton reaction, catalyzed by transition metal ions like ferrous iron and cuprous copper, is the key pathway for generating the highly toxic hydroxyl radical [25, 76]. Therefore, specifically chelating these catalytic metal ions can fundamentally suppress the initiation of the free radical chain reaction.

Iron chelators, such as deferiprone and deferoxamine, work by efficiently binding free iron. This prevents its participation in the Fenton reaction, thereby reducing hydroxyl radical production. This strategy shows promise in neurodegenerative disease research, suggesting potential application for the similarly vulnerable auditory neural system [76, 77]. Future development may involve optimizing the inner ear targeting of chelators and exploring synergistic combinations with other agents, like NAC. The goal is to enhance protection for spiral ganglion neurons while reducing side effects [77]. Research on specific oxidative damage pathways also suggests new directions. For instance, in a cochlear explant culture model, exogenous NAD + prevented neuroaxonal and hair cell degeneration induced by mefloquine or manganese. It achieved this by inhibiting caspase-3-dependent apoptosis. This finding informs targeted protection strategies based on energy metabolism and apoptosis regulation [78–80]. A more advanced concept involves designing multifunctional targeted antioxidants. One example is chemically linking an anti-inflammatory drug, such as an NSAID, with a potent antioxidant moiety like Trolox. This creates a novel molecule possessing dual anti-inflammatory and antioxidant functions [80]. Such designs may not only enhance bioactivity but also improve drug properties through structural modification. Although currently designed for conditions like atherosclerosis, the core principle of multi-target, synergistic action offers important insights for inner ear drug development. Notably, novel oral multifunctional antioxidants designed for inner ear diseases have shown significant preventive effects in animal models. They protect against noise-induced hearing loss [81] and the loss of hair cells and spiral ganglion neurons caused by blast shockwaves [82]. These results lay a solid foundation for future translational research.

7. Conclusion

This article systematically demonstrates that antioxidant therapy for sensorineural hearing loss can be harmful if applied indiscriminately or excessively. Such an approach may damage inner ear hair cells and spiral ganglion neurons. The normal function of the inner ear depends on a precisely regulated redox homeostasis. Exogenous antioxidant interventions applied without precise guidance are unlikely to effectively terminate free radical chain reactions. Instead, they risk disrupting physiological reactive oxygen species signaling, inducing an "antioxidant paradox," and even catalyzing the generation of more toxic hydroxyl radicals. This disrupts homeostasis and exacerbates cellular damage. Future therapeutic strategies must shift from a broad-cavenging approach to one of precise modulation. Key priorities include developing non-invasive technologies for diagnosing oxidative stress directly within the inner ear. Furthermore, exploring novel strategies is essential. These include selective neutralization using hydrogen, source blockade via metal ion chelation, and multifunctional targeted drug delivery. The core objective should be to restore and maintain the inner ear's intrinsic redox balance, rather than blindly combating all free radicals. Only this focused approach can safely and effectively advance the prevention and treatment of hearing loss.

Acknowledgments

The authors gratefully acknowledge the financial support from the National Natural Science Foundation of China (82,371,158 and 82,071,050).

Conflict of interest

The authors declare no conflict of interest.

Author details

Liling Li[1], Dalian Ding[2] and Peng Li[1]*

1 Department of Otolaryngology, Head and Neck Surgery, The Third Affiliated Hospital of Sun Yat-Sen University, Guang Zhou, China

2 State University of New York at Buffalo, New York, USA

*Address all correspondence to: lipeng25@mail.sysu.edu.cn

References

[1] Teraoka M, Hato N, Inufusa H, You F. Role of oxidative stress in sensorineural hearing loss. International Journal of Molecular Sciences. 2024;**25**(8):4146. DOI: 10.3390/ijms25084146

[2] Maniaci A, La Via L, Lechien JR, et al. Hearing loss and Oxidative Stress: A comprehensive review. Antioxidants (Basel). 2024;**13**(7):842. DOI: 10.3390/antiox13070842

[3] Nunez DA, Guo RC. Acquired sensorineural hearing loss, oxidative stress, and microRNAs. Neural Regeneration Research. 2025;**20**(9):2513–2519. DOI: 10.3724/abbs.2022018

[4] Kishimoto-Urata M, Urata S, Fujimoto C, Yamasoba T. Role of oxidative stress and antioxidants in acquired Inner Ear Disorders. Antioxidants (Basel). 2022;**11**(8):1469. DOI: 10.3390/antiox11081469

[5] Meng L, Liu S, Luo J, et al. Oxidative stress and reactive oxygen species in otorhinolaryngological diseases: Insights from pathophysiology to targeted antioxidant therapies. Redox Report. 2025;**30**(1):2458942. DOI: 10.1080/13510002.2025.2458942

[6] McFadden SL, Ding D, Burkard RF, et al. Cu/Zn SOD deficiency potentiates hearing loss and cochlear pathology in aged 129,CD-1 mice. The Journal of Comparative Neurology 1999;**413**:101–112

[7] McFadden SL, Ding D, Reaume AG, Flood DG, Salvi RJ. Age-related cochlear hair cell loss is enhanced in mice lacking copper/zinc superoxide dismutase. Neurobiology of Aging. 1999;**20**(1):1–8. DOI: 10.1016/s0197-4580(99)00018-4

[8] McFadden SL, Ding D, Ohlemiller K, Salvi R. The role of superoxide dismutase in Age-related and noise-induced hearing Loss: Clues from SOD1 knockout mice. Florida: James F Willott Handbook of Mouse Auditory Research CRS Press; 2001. 1489–1504 p. DOI: 10.1201/9781420038736-40

[9] McFadden SL, Ohlemiller KK, Ding D, Shero M, Salvi RJ.The influence of superoxide dismutase and glutathione peroxidase deficiencies on noise-induced hearing loss in Mice. Noise & Health. 2001;**3**(11):49–64

[10] Han C, Kim MJ, Ding D, et al. GSR is not essential for the maintenance of antioxidant defenses in mouse cochlea: Possible role of the thioredoxin system as a functional backup for GSR. PLoS One. 2017;**12**(7):e0180817. DOI: 10.1371/journal.pone.0180817

[11] Jeong M, Kurihara S, Stankovic KM. An in Vitro oxidative stress model of the Human Inner Ear using human-induced pluripotent stem cell-derived otic progenitor cells. Antioxidants (Basel). 2024;**13**(11):1407. DOI: 10.3390/antiox13111407

[12] Pak JH, Kim Y, Yi J, Chung JW. Antioxidant therapy against oxidative damage of the Inner Ear: Protection and preconditioning. Antioxidants (Basel). 2020;**9**(11):1076. DOI: 10.3390/antiox9111076

[13] Lin X, Li L, Luo J, et al. Cobalt-induced apoptosis of cochlear organotypic cultures and HEI-OC1 cells

is mediated by Dicer. Neurotoxicology. 2024;**100**:85–99

[14] Su Z, Chen Y, Liu Y, et al. Oxidative stress and inflammation combine to exacerbate cochlear damage and sensorineural hearing loss in C57BL/6 mice. Frontiers in Neuroscience. 2025;**19**:1563428. DOI: 10.3389/fnins.2025.1563428

[15] Shih CP, Kuo CY, Lin YY, et al. Inhibition of Cochlear HMGB1 expression attenuates oxidative stress and inflammation in an experimental Murine Model of Noise-Induced hearing loss. Cells. 2021;**10**(4):810. DOI: 10.3390/cells10040810

[16] Mastino P, Rosati D, de Soccio G, et al. Oxidative stress in obstructive sleep Apnea syndrome: Putative pathways to hearing system impairment. Antioxidants (Basel). 2023;**12**(7):1430. DOI: 10.3390/antiox12071430

[17] Di Paola R, Siracusa R, Fusco R, et al. Redox modulation of meniere disease by Coriolus versicolor Treatment, a nutritional mushroom approach with neuroprotective potential. Current Neuropharmacology. 2024;**22**(12):2079–2098. DOI: 10.2174/1570159X22666231206153936

[18] American Diabetes Association Professional Practice Committee. 2. Diagnosis and classification of diabetes: Standards of care in Diabetes-2025. Diabetes Care. 2025;**48**(Suppl Supplement_1):S27–S49. DOI: 10.2337/dc25-S002

[19] Gentilin E, Cani A, Simoni E, et al. Hydrogen peroxide toxicity on auditory cells: An in vitro study. Chemico-Biological Interactions. 2021;**345**:109575. 109575. DOI: 10.1016/j.cbi.2021.109575

[20] Suzuki Y, Hayashi K, Goto F, et al. Premature senescence is regulated by crosstalk among TFEB, the autophagy lysosomal pathway and ROS derived from damaged mitochondria in NaAsO2-exposed auditory cells. Cell Death Discovery. 2024;**10**(1):382. DOI: 10.1038/s41420-024-02139-4

[21] Li J, Dai X, He X, et al. Effect of SOD2 methylation on mitochondrial DNA4834-bp deletion mutation in marginal cells under oxidative stress. Bosnian Journal of Basic Medical Sciences. 2020;**20**(1):70–77. DOI: 10.17305/bjbms.2019.4353

[22] Wan H, Chen H, Liu J, et al. PARP1 inhibition prevents oxidative stress in age-related hearing loss via PAR-Ca2+-AIF axis in cochlear strial marginal cells. Free Radical Biology and Medicine. 2024;**220**:222–235

[23] Xie W, Shu T, Peng H, et al. LncRNA H19 inhibits oxidative stress injury of cochlear hair cells by regulating miR-653-5p/SIRT1 axis. Acta Biochimica Et Biophysica Sinica. 2022;**54**(3):332–339. DOI: 10.3724/abbs.2022018

[24] Chandimali N, Bak SG, Park EH, et al. Free radicals and their impact on health and antioxidant defenses: A review. Cell Death Discovery. 2025;**11**(1):19. DOI: 10.1038/s41420-024-02278-8

[25] Zhao Z. Hydroxyl radical generations form the physiologically relevant Fenton-like reactions. Free Radical Biology and Medicine. 2023;**208**:510–515. DOI: 10.1016/j.freeradbiomed.2023.09.013

[26] Wang C, Wang Z, Zeng B, et al. Fenton-like reaction of the iron(II)-histidine complex generates hydroxyl radicals: Implications for oxidative

stress and Alzheimer's disease. Chemical Communications. 2021;**57**(92):12293–12296. DOI: 10.1039/d1cc05000a

[27] Keshtkar Vanashi A, Ghasemzadeh H. Copper(II) containing chitosan hydrogel as a heterogeneous Fenton-like catalyst for production of hydroxyl radical: A quantitative study. International Journal of Biological Macromolecules. 2022;**199**:348–357. DOI: 10.1016/j.ijbiomac.2021.12.150

[28] Selyutina OY, Babenko SV, Slepneva IA, Polyakov NE, Kontoghiorghes GJ. Increased Free Radical Generation during the Interaction of a Quinone-Quinoline Chelator with Metal Ions and the Enhancing Effect of Light. Pharmaceuticals. 2023;**16**(8):1116. DOI: 10.3390/ph16081116

[29] Unsal V, Cicek M, İ S. Toxicity of carbon tetrachloride, free radicals and role of antioxidants. Reviews on Environmental Health. 2020;**36**(2):279–295. DOI: 10.1515/reveh-2020-0048

[30] Korovesis D, Rubio-Tomás T, Tavernarakis N. Oxidative stress in Age-Related neurodegenerative diseases: An Overview of Recent Tools and Findings. Antioxidants (Basel). 2023;**12**(1):131. DOI: 10.3390/antiox12010131

[31] Gebicki JM, Nauser T. Initiation and prevention of biological damage by Radiation-Generated protein radicals. International Journal of Molecular Sciences. 2021;**23**(1):396. DOI: 10.3390/ijms23010396

[32] Wang L, Ding D, Salvi R, Roth JA. Nicotinamide adenine dinucleotide prevents neuroaxonal degeneration induced by manganese in cochlear organotypic cultures. Neurotoxicology. 2014;**40**:65–74. DOI: 10.1016/j.neuro.2013.11.007

[33] Ding D, Zhang J, Liu F, et al. Antioxidative stress-induced damage in cochlear explants. Journal of Otology. 2020;**15**(1):36–40. DOI: 10.1016/j.joto.2019.11.005

[34] Li L, Chen D, Lin X, et al. Antioxidative Stress-Induced destruction to cochlear cells caused by blind antioxidant therapy. Otolaryngology–Head and Neck Surgery. 2024;**00**(0). DOI: 10.1002/ohn.659

[35] Gallo-Cordova A, Nuñez N, Díaz-Ufano C, et al. Insights into the formation of free radicals using metal ferrite nanocatalysts (MFe2O4, M=Fe, Mn, Zn, Co) prepared by a highly reproducible microwave-assisted polyol method. Nanoscale. 2025;**17**(33):19182–19195. DOI: 10.1039/d5nr02101d

[36] Duan M, Zhu Z, Pi H, et al. Mechanistic Insights and Analytical Advances in Food Antioxidants: A comprehensive review of molecular pathways, detection technologies, and nutritional applications. Antioxidants (Basel). 2025;**14**(4):438. DOI: 10.3390/antiox14040438

[37] Ghaedamini H, Kim DS. Recent advances in electrochemical detection of reactive oxygen species: A review. Analyst. 2025;**150**(8):1490–1517. DOI: 10.1039/d4an01533a

[38] Jamshidi M, Walcarius A, Thangamuthu M, Mehrgardi M, Ranjbar A. Electrochemical approaches based on micro- and nanomaterials for diagnosing oxidative stress. Microchimica Acta. 2023;**190**(4):117. DOI: 10.1007/s00604-023-05681-7

[39] Munteanu IG, Apetrei C. A review on electrochemical sensors and biosensors used in assessing antioxidant activity. Antioxidants (Basel). 2022;**11** (3):584. DOI: 10.3390/antiox11030584

[40] Cao X, Liu T, Wang X, et al. Recent advances in nanozyme-based sensing technology for antioxidant detection. Sensors. 2024;**24**(20):6616. DOI: 10.3390/s24206616

[41] Zhang Y, Sigaeva A, Elías-Llumbet A, et al. Free radical detection in precision-cut mouse liver slices with diamond-based quantum sensing. Proceedings of the National Academy of Sciences of the United States of America. 2024;**121**(43):e2317921121. DOI: 10.1073/pnas.2317921121

[42] Mendonça JDS, Guimarães RCA, Zorgetto-Pinheiro VA, et al. Natural antioxidant evaluation: A review of detection Methods. Molecules. 2022;**27** (11):3563. DOI: 10.3390/molecules27113563

[43] Ashok A, Andrabi SS, Mansoor S, et al. Antioxidant therapy in oxidative Stress-induced Neurodegenerative diseases: Role of nanoparticle-based drug delivery systems in clinical translation. Antioxidants (Basel). 2022;**11**(2):408. DOI: 10.3390/antiox11020408

[44] Pappolla MA, Martins RN, Poeggeler B, Omar RA, Perry G. Oxidative stress in Alzheimer's Disease: The shortcomings of antioxidant therapies. Journal of Alzheimer's Disease. 2024;**101**(s1):S155–S178. DOI: 10.3233/JAD-240659

[45] Hajmohammadi Z, Bagher Z, Taghizadeh-Hesary F, et al. Nanodelivery of antioxidant Agents: A promising strategy for preventing sensorineural hearing loss. European Journal of Pharmaceutics and Biopharmaceutics. 2024;**202**:114393. DOI: 10.1016/j.ejpb.2024.114393

[46] Harris IS, DeNicola GM. The Complex Interplay between Antioxidants and ROS in Cancer. Trends in Cell Biology. 2020;**30**(6):440–451. DOI: 10.1016/j.tcb.2020.03.002

[47] Malcangi G, Patano A, Ciocia AM, et al. Benefits of Natural Antioxidants on Oral Health. Antioxidants (Basel). 2023;**12**(6):1309. DOI: 10.3390/antiox12061309

[48] Halliwell B. Understanding mechanisms of antioxidant action in health and disease. Nature Reviews Molecular Cell Biology. 2024;**25**(1):13–33. DOI: 10.1038/s41580-023-00645-4

[49] Nam YE, Kim HJ, Kwon O. Acute and prolonged effects of Bacillus amyloliquefaciens GF424-derived SOD on antioxidant defense in healthy individuals challenged with intense aerobic exercise. Free Radical Biology and Medicine. 2024;**224**:484–493. DOI: 10.1016/j.freeradbiomed.2024.09.015

[50] Yoshikawa T, You F. Oxidative stress and bio-regulation. International Journal of Molecular Sciences. 2024;**25** (6):3360. DOI: 10.3390/ijms25063360

[51] McFadden SL, Ding D, Salvemini D, Salvi RJ. M40403, a superoxide dismutase mimetic, protects cochlear hair cells from gentamicin, but not cisplatin toxicity. Toxicology and Applied Pharmacology. 2003;**186**(1):46–54. DOI: 10.1016/s0041-008x(02)00017-0

[52] Nicotera TM, Ding D, McFadden SL, Salvemini D, Salvi R. Paraquat-induced hair cell damage and

protection with the superoxide dismutase mimetic m40403. Audiology and Neurotology. 2004;**9**(6):353–362. DOI: 10.1159/000081284

[53] Anik MI, Mahmud N, Masud AA, et al. Role of reactive oxygen species in aging and age-related diseases: A review. ACS Applied Bio Materials. 2022;**5**:4028–4054

[54] Rusciano D, Bagnoli P. Oxygen, the paradox of life and the eye. Frontiers in Bioscience-Landmark. 2024;**29**(9):319. DOI: 10.3390/ijms25063360

[55] Deng L, Ding D, Su J, Manohar S, Salvi R. Salicylate selectively kills cochlear spiral ganglion neurons by paradoxically up-regulating superoxide. Neurotoxicity Research. 2013;**24**(3):307–319. DOI: 10.1016/S0041-008X(02)00017-0

[56] White K, Kim MJ, Han C, et al. Loss of IDH2 accelerates age-related hearing loss in male mice. Scientific Reports. 2018;**8**(1):5039. DOI: 10.1038/s41598-018-23436-w

[57] McFadden SL, Woo JM, Michalak N, Ding D. Dietary vitamin C supplementation reduces noise-induced hearing loss in Guinea pigs. Hearing Research. 2005;**202**(1-2):200–208. DOI: 10.1016/j.heares.2004.10.011

[58] Ding D, Jiang H, Chen GD, et al. N-acetyl-cysteine prevents age-related hearing loss and the progressive loss of inner hair cells in γ-glutamyl transferase 1 deficient mice. Aging. 2016;**8**(4):730–750. DOI: 10.1021/acsabm.2c00411

[59] Liu Y, Wu G, Feng L, et al. Harnessing antioxidants in cancer therapy: Opportunities, challenges, and future directions. Antioxidants (Basel). 2025;**14**(6):674. DOI: 10.3390/antiox14060674

[60] Kilicarslan You D, Fuwad A, Lee KH, et al. Evaluation of the protective role of Vitamin E against ROS-Driven lipid oxidation in model cell membranes. Antioxidants (Basel). 2024;**13**(9):1135. DOI: 10.3390/antiox13091135

[61] Çelik EE, Gökmen V. Interactions between free and bound antioxidants under different conditions in food systems. Critical Reviews in Food Science and Nutrition. 2022;**62**(21):5766–5782. DOI: 10.1080/10408398.2021.1892584

[62] Nikolaidis MG, Margaritelis NV. Free radicals and antioxidants: Appealing to magic. Trends in Endocrinology & Metabolism. 2023;**34**(9):503–504. DOI: 10.1016/j.tem.2023.06.001

[63] Bjelakovic G, Nikolova D, Simonetti RG, Gluud C. Antioxidant supplements for prevention of gastrointestinal cancers: A systematic review and meta-analysis. The Lancet. 2004;**364**(9441):1219–1228. DOI: 10.1016/S0140-6736(04)17138-9

[64] Bjelakovic G, Nikolova D, Gluud LL, Simonetti RG, Gluud C. Mortality in randomized trials of antioxidant supplements for primary and secondary prevention: Systematic review and meta-analysis. JAMA. 2007;**297**(8):842–857. DOI: 10.1001/jama.297.8.842

[65] Villanueva C, Kross RD. Antioxidant-induced stress. International Journal of Molecular Sciences. 2012;**13**(2):2091–2109. DOI: 10.3390/ijms13022091

[66] Poljsak B, Milisav I. The neglected significance of "antioxidative stress". Oxidative Medicine and Cellular Longevity. 2012;**2012**:480895. DOI: 10.1155/2012/480895

[67] Dündar Y, Aslan R. Antioxidative stress. Eastern Journal of Medicine. 2000;**5**:45–47

[68] Halliwell B. Free radicals and antioxidants: Updating a personal view. Nutrition Reviews. 2012;**70**(5):257–265. DOI: 10.1111/j.1753-4887.2012.00476.x

[69] WANG L, Dalian DING, Hong SUN, et al. Introspection of oxidant/antioxidant imbalance in the inner ear. Journal of Clinical Otorhinolaryngology Head and Neck Surgery. 2013;**27**(17):965–974. DOI: 10.13201/j.issn.1001-1781.2013.17.018

[70] Ohta S. Molecular hydrogen as a preventive and therapeutic medical gas: Initiation, development and potential of hydrogen medicine. Pharmacology & Therapeutics. 2014;**144**(1):1–11. DOI: 10.1016/j.pharmthera.2014.04.006

[71] Ichihara M, Sobue S, Ito M, et al. Beneficial biological effects and the underlying mechanisms of molecular hydrogen - comprehensive review of 321 original articles. Medical Gas Research. 2015;**5**:12

[72] Johnsen HM, Hiorth M, Klaveness J. Molecular hydrogen therapy-A Review on clinical studies and outcomes. Molecules. 2023;**28**(23):7785. DOI: 10.3390/molecules28237785

[73] Dhillon G, Buddhavarapu V, Grewal H, et al. Hydrogen water: Extra healthy or a Hoax?-A systematic review. International Journal of Molecular Sciences. 2024;**25**(2):973. DOI: 10.3390/ijms25020973

[74] Zhang Y, Fan W, Li X, Wang WX, Liu S. Enhanced removal of free radicals by aqueous Hydrogen nanobubbles and their role in oxidative stress. Environmental Science & Technology. 2022;**56**(21):15096–15107. DOI: 10.1021/acs.est.2c03707

[75] Koyama Y, Kobayashi Y, Kobayashi H, Shimada S. Diverse possibilities of SI-Based agent, A unique new antioxidant. Antioxidants (Basel). 2023;**12**(5):1061. DOI: 10.3390/antiox12051061

[76] Halliwell B. Reflections of an aging free radical. Free Radical Biology and Medicine. 2020;**161**:234–245. DOI: 10.1016/j.freeradbiomed.2020.10.010

[77] Kontoghiorghes GJ. New approaches and strategies for the repurposing of Iron Chelating/Antioxidant drugs for diseases of free radical Pathology in Medicine. Antioxidants (Basel). 2025;**14**(8):982. DOI: 10.3390/antiox14080982

[78] Ding D, Qi W, Yu D, et al. Addition of exogenous NAD+ prevents mefloquine-induced neuroaxonal and hair cell degeneration through reduction of caspase-3-mediated apoptosis in cochlear organotypic cultures. PLoS One. 2013;**8**(11):e79817. DOI: 10.1371/journal.pone.0079817

[79] Ding D, Jiang H, Fu Y, et al. Ototoxic model of oxaliplatin and protection from Nicotinamide Adenine Dinucleotide. Journal of Otology. 2013;**8**(1):63–71. DOI: 10.1371/journal.pone.0079817

[80] Tzara A, Lambrinidis G, Kourounakis A. Design of Multifaceted

antioxidants: Shifting towards Anti-Inflammatory and Antihyperlipidemic activity. Molecules. 2021;**26**(16):4928. DOI: 10.3390/molecules26164928

[81] Chen GD, Daszynski DM, Ding D, et al. Novel oral multifunctional antioxidant prevents noise-induced hearing loss and hair cell loss. Hearing Research. 2020;**388**:107880. DOI: 10.1016/j.heares.2019.107880

[82] Ding D, Manohar S, Kador PF, Salvi R. Multifunctional redox modulator prevents blast-induced loss of cochlear and vestibular hair cells and auditory spiral ganglion neurons. Scientific Reports. 2024;**14**(1):15296. DOI: 10.1038/s41598-024-66406-1

Section 3

Clinical Evaluation and Correlations

Chapter 4

Cognitive Decline and Hearing Loss: The Importance of Assessment

Rochele Martins Machado, Karina Carlesso Pagliarin and Fernanda Soares Aurélio Patatt

Abstract

Hearing loss significantly compromises communication, social interaction, and multiple dimensions of quality of life. Furthermore, it is associated with an increased risk of cognitive decline, affecting processes such as memory, attention, language, and executive functions. The cognitive overload imposed by the effort required to understand speech in unfavorable acoustic conditions may anticipate or intensify neurodegenerative processes, particularly in older adults. Added to this is the impact of social isolation, reduced autonomy, and decreased participation in cognitively stimulating activities—factors that may mediate or accelerate this decline. In this context, the use of specific tools to assess cognition in individuals with hearing loss becomes essential, as tests that rely exclusively on the auditory modality tend to underestimate actual performance, leading to biased interpretations. To support healthcare professionals, particularly those in Speech-Language Pathology, Audiology, and Neuropsychology, this chapter presents the relationship between hearing loss and cognition, highlighting mechanisms, explanatory hypotheses, and recent epidemiological evidence. It also describes the instruments traditionally used in cognitive assessment and provides an in-depth discussion of specific tools developed or adapted for individuals with hearing impairment, introducing the Montreal Cognitive Assessment for Hearing Impairment (MoCA-H) as an appropriate instrument for these cases. By presenting these approaches, the chapter reinforces the importance of more precise assessment strategies that allow for reliable diagnoses, early identification of cognitive changes, and the planning of effective interventions. In doing so, it contributes to improving clinical practice and promoting integrated care that jointly considers both auditory and cognitive health.

Keywords: hearing disorder, cognition, cognitive screening test, cognitive decline, hearing loss

1. Introduction

Hearing loss ranks among the most disabling chronic conditions, affecting communication, functionality, and social participation, while also representing a significant global public health challenge [1]. Approximately 430 million adults worldwide are estimated to experience some degree of hearing loss, underscoring its epidemiological magnitude and potential impact on quality of life [2].

In addition to restricting social interaction, hearing loss results in a range of communicative and cognitive impairments [3]. Scientific evidence demonstrates a strong association between untreated hearing loss and cognitive decline [4–7]. It is considered the most significant potentially modifiable midlife risk factor for the development of dementia [8]. Hearing loss contributes to neural system deterioration and reduced brain function [9, 10]. Furthermore, the acceleration of cognitive decline may stem from social isolation, reduced communication, and loss of autonomy – factors frequently associated with hearing loss [11–13].

Given these concerns, it is essential that individuals with hearing loss undergo evaluation to determine the impact of this condition on cognitive processes. This requires the adoption of cognitive assessment strategies that account for and minimize biases introduced by hearing loss. Instruments relying exclusively on oral instructions and auditory input tend to underestimate an individual's actual cognitive performance, thereby increasing the risk of misdiagnosis [14].

Accordingly, the use of visual or multimodal versions of cognitive tests – specifically designed and validated for individuals with hearing loss – is strongly recommended. Likewise, the routine integration of standardized sensory assessments into the diagnostic process is critical to ensure greater accuracy and reliability in the interpretation of clinical results [15].

In this context, the present chapter provides an updated synthesis of the literature on the relationship between hearing loss and cognitive changes, highlighting the main scientific evidence available. It also reviews the cognitive assessments most commonly employed in clinical practice and discusses specific instruments and protocols developed or adapted for individuals with hearing loss, with the aim of guiding professionals and researchers in selecting the most appropriate and reliable methods for this population.

2. Hearing loss and cognitive impairments

Untreated hearing loss has significant effects on cognition across different stages of life, regardless of age. Growing evidence demonstrates that prolonged auditory deprivation compromises neural stimulation and may accelerate processes of brain reorganization, overloading cognitive resources required for speech comprehension and attention maintenance [6–16]. This redirection of cognitive effort negatively affects functions such as memory, language, and executive abilities, fostering mental overload and cognitive fatigue [16]. In addition, communication difficulties contribute to social isolation, reduced participation in intellectual activities, and lower engagement in meaningful interactions – factors recognized as potential mediators of cognitive decline [17–19]. Thus, the early detection and management of hearing loss should be understood as essential measures not only for preserving communication but also for promoting cognitive health at all ages.

In midlife, hearing loss has been widely recognized as one of the main modifiable risk factors for cognitive decline and the development of dementia [8]. In the Brazilian context, data from a longitudinal study showed that individuals with elevated hearing thresholds experienced a faster decline in global cognitive performance over eight years, even after controlling for socioeconomic and lifestyle variables [20]. Similarly, a long-term international investigation identified a dose–response effect between elevated hearing thresholds and cognitive decline over more than two decades of follow-up, reinforcing the hypothesis of a plausible causal link [21].

Similarly, presbycusis – age-related hearing loss – is one of the most prevalent chronic conditions in the elderly population, representing a multifactorial phenomenon of natural aging. From a pathophysiological perspective, it involves progressive degenerative changes in both the peripheral and central auditory systems, including the loss of cochlear hair cells, degeneration of neural auditory pathways, and biochemical and metabolic alterations. These changes impair sound detection and discrimination, resulting in speech comprehension difficulties, particularly in acoustically challenging environments, which are associated with cognitive overload and an increased risk of cognitive decline and dementia [8, 22].

The relationship between presbycusis and cognitive decline has been explained by several etiological hypotheses. These include the cognitive load hypothesis, which suggests that the continuous effort required to understand speech in adverse conditions reduces the resources available for other cognitive functions; the common cause hypothesis, which proposes shared neurodegenerative or vascular mechanisms; and the cascade hypothesis, which emphasizes the roles of sensory deprivation and social isolation in accelerating cognitive decline. Additionally, evidence indicates that hearing loss may serve as an early marker of ongoing neurodegenerative processes [23].

Studies indicate that a 10 dB reduction in hearing acuity is associated with decreased cognitive function and a higher risk of developing dementia [4, 5, 7, 24]. Moreover, even subclinical hearing loss, with thresholds below 25 dB, has been linked to deficits in attention, memory, and processing speed, suggesting that cognitive changes may arise before the formal diagnosis of hearing loss [4].

Accordingly, auditory rehabilitation through the use of hearing aids has shown consistent positive effects on cognition in adults and older adults with hearing loss. Evidence from longitudinal studies and clinical trials indicates that adequate sound amplification contributes to the maintenance or improvement of cognitive performance, including attention, memory, and executive functions, while also reducing the risk of cognitive decline and dementia. These benefits appear to result both from reduced cognitive overload associated with impaired auditory perception and from enhanced social participation and effective communication. Thus, auditory intervention not only restores hearing function but also indirectly contributes to preserving cognitive health, underscoring the importance of early detection of hearing loss and the adoption of personalized auditory rehabilitation strategies [25–29].

3. Cognitive assessments

Cognitive assessment is an essential tool for understanding higher mental functions, including memory, attention, language, executive functions, perception, and reasoning. Through standardized instruments, it is possible to identify alterations that impact an individual's functionality, contributing to clinical diagnoses, therapeutic planning, and the monitoring of neurological and psychiatric disease progression [30, 31]. Moreover, in the context of population aging, cognitive assessment becomes even more relevant as it enables the early detection of mild cognitive impairment and dementia, supporting timely interventions and rehabilitation strategies [8, 32–34].

The appropriate choice of instrument is fundamental to ensuring sensitivity and specificity, avoiding false negatives, and enabling more targeted therapeutic planning. Methodological advances have improved diagnostic precision and fostered the development of personalized interventions in both clinical care and research at the interface of cognition and hearing. Accordingly, different instruments have been developed to assess cognition, organized according to their main objectives and target populations. The following section briefly presents the tools most commonly used in clinical practice.

Among the cognitive screening tests applied to the general population, the Mini-Mental State Examination (MMSE) [35], the Montreal Cognitive Assessment (MoCA) [36], and the Alzheimer's Disease Assessment Scale – Cognitive Subscale (ADAS-Cog) [37] are widely used for screening and monitoring cognitive decline. To investigate executive and frontal functions, the most commonly employed instruments include the Frontal Assessment Battery (FAB) [38], the Stroop Test [39], and the Wisconsin Card Sorting Test (WCST) [40], which assess processes such as inhibition, flexibility, and planning. In the field of memory, the Rey Auditory Verbal Learning Test (RAVLT) [41] and the Wechsler Memory Scale (WMS) [42] stand out, both addressing different modalities of episodic and working memory. Attention and processing speed can be examined with the Trail Making Test (TMT-A and TMT-B) [43] and the Digit Span [44], which provide objective measures of attentional performance. Regarding language, the most widely used instruments are the Boston Naming Test (BNT) [45], designed to assess confrontational naming, and the Token Test [46], which investigates verbal comprehension of commands. Finally, the Cambridge Neuropsychological Test Automated Battery (CANTAB) [47–49] is a computerized, visual, non-verbal tool sensitive to subtle cognitive deficits.

Among the most widely used screening tools, the MMSE has become one of the most applied instruments for older adults and patients with suspected dementia worldwide. Administration takes an average of 5–10 minutes and assesses orientation, memory, attention, calculation, language, and constructive praxis, with a maximum score of 30 points. Importantly, score interpretation must take into account the educational level of the individual, as it directly influences performance [35].

Complementing the MMSE, the MoCA was developed to overcome its limitations, particularly in detecting mild cognitive impairment. Administration takes an average of 10–15 minutes and covers eight domains: attention and concentration, executive functions, memory, language, visuospatial skills, abstraction, delayed recall, and orientation, with a maximum score of 30 points. A score below 26 indicates possible cognitive impairment, and one point should be added to the total score for individuals with up to 12 years of formal education to minimize educational bias. The MoCA is recommended for adults and older adults under investigation for cognitive decline, being particularly useful in the early stages of dementia but also applicable in neurological conditions such as Parkinson's disease, stroke, and multiple sclerosis. Its high sensitivity and ease of use have established it as one of the most recommended tools for early cognitive screening [36]. Currently, 86 MoCA versions have been adapted to different cultural contexts, including English, French, Arabic, Chinese, German, and Dutch, among others [50]. In Brazil, the MoCA-BR was translated, adapted, and validated for the Brazilian cultural and linguistic context, preserving the original structure for evaluating multiple cognitive domains [51]. National studies have demonstrated its utility in older adults, particularly for screening mild cognitive impairment and early dementia [52, 53]. The cutoff generally adopted in Brazil is ≤ 25 points to indicate possible impairment, although validation studies have shown variations depending on the sample analyzed [51]. As in the original version, one point should be added for individuals with up to 12 years of education. Thus, the MoCA-BR has been consolidated as a reliable and sensitive tool for cognitive screening in the Brazilian clinical context, expanding its applicability in both research and practice.

Another widely used instrument is the ADAS-Cog, applied extensively to assess the progression of Alzheimer's disease. It has a significant impact in both specialized clinical practice and clinical trials of new treatments, where it is recognized as the gold standard for measuring cognitive outcomes. Administration takes an average of 30–45 minutes and includes tasks involving memory, language, praxis, and attention, providing a detailed profile of cognitive performance [37].

In the field of executive functions, the FAB was designed as a brief and practical measure of frontal lobe executive abilities. It comprises six subtests and can be administered in approximately 10 minutes at the bedside. Developed for use in adults and older adults, it is particularly useful in clinical and research contexts investigating frontal syndromes and neurodegenerative diseases [38]. The demand for culturally adapted tools led to the development of the Brazilian version (BAF), which underwent translation, back-translation, and expert review to ensure conceptual equivalence with the original version. The BAF retained the six-subtest structure, preserving its brevity and clinical applicability, and demonstrated good internal consistency, high inter-rater reliability, and discriminant validity for differentiating controls from patients with frontal syndromes. Thus, the Brazilian version reinforced the clinical utility of the instrument in national contexts, extending its applicability to hospital, outpatient, and research settings while maintaining the essential characteristics of the original study [54].

Another widely applied test in adults and older adults, also used with adolescents and various clinical populations – including dementia, frontal lobe lesions, Parkinson's disease, attention-deficit/hyperactivity disorder (ADHD), and schizophrenia – is the Stroop Test. It has become a robust measure of selective attention, inhibitory control, processing speed, and cognitive flexibility, and remains one of the most influential experimental paradigms in cognitive psychology and clinical neuropsychology [39]. Stroop experiments demonstrated that automatic word reading strongly interferes with the task of naming the ink color in which the words are printed. This interference results in longer reaction times and more errors when word and color are incongruent (e.g., the word "red" written in blue ink), an effect that persists even after repetition and practice.

The WCST is another widely used protocol for adults and older adults, also applicable to adolescents and clinical populations with frontal lobe dysfunction, such as traumatic brain injury, Parkinson's disease, schizophrenia, ADHD, and various dementias [40]. In the original experiments, participants classified cards according to varying criteria (color, shape, or number), and after successive correct responses, the categorization rule was changed without warning, requiring strategic adjustments based on feedback. The WCST has been established as a robust tool for assessing abstract reasoning, concept formation, cognitive flexibility, and executive functions, as performance is characterized by the ability to shift strategies in response to changing rules, with perseverative errors reflecting difficulties in cognitive flexibility.

The RAVLT, originally developed by André Rey in 1941 and later consolidated in L'examen clinique en psychologie [41], is one of the most widely used instruments for assessing verbal episodic memory. It is highly recognized in the neuropsychological literature for measuring learning, immediate and delayed recall, and recognition. The test also allows for the analysis of intrusions, perseverations, false positive/negative errors, susceptibility to interference, and short-term memory indicators [55, 56]. The RAVLT uses List A with 15 words presented across five trials (A1–A5) to evaluate learning, followed by an interference list (List B, B1), immediate recall of List A (A6), delayed recall after 20–30 minutes (A7), and finally a recognition test. It is applicable to adolescents, adults, and older adults, in both research and clinical practice, and is particularly useful for assessing verbal memory deficits in pathological aging and dementia [57].

The Wechsler Memory Scale (WMS), developed by American psychologist David Wechsler, is one of the most traditional and widely used instruments in both clinical and research contexts [42]. Initially applied to hospitalized adults, it has since expanded across successive revisions to include populations ranging from adolescents to older adults (16–90 years). The WMS provides a comprehensive assessment of different memory aspects, including auditory memory, visual memory, working memory, immediate recall, and delayed recall, offering specific indices that aid in the differential diagnosis of neurological and psychiatric conditions such as dementia, traumatic brain injury, and affective disorders. With successive revisions, now culminating in the WMS-IV, the instrument remains an international benchmark, widely applied in both clinical and research contexts, and is regarded as a milestone in standardized memory assessment [58].

The TMT, composed of Parts A (TMT-A) and B (TMT-B), originated in the United States as part of the Army Individual Test Battery [43]. It has become widely used in both clinical and research neuropsychology. TMT-A evaluates sustained attention, processing speed, and visuomotor coordination through sequential number connections, while TMT-B requires alternating between numbers and letters, demanding greater cognitive flexibility and executive control. Performance on the TMT is strongly influenced by sociodemographic variables, especially age and education, which must be considered when interpreting results [59].

The Digit Span subtest is one of the most widely used international measures in neuropsychological assessment, designed to evaluate attention, short-term memory, and auditory working memory [44]. The task involves orally presented random number sequences delivered by the examiner at one-second intervals. The participant must repeat them in different conditions: in forward order, to assess attention and immediate retention; and in backward order, requiring greater working memory engagement. Each item consists of two trials with sequences of the same length but different numbers, with increasing difficulty [60]. The Digit Span is broadly applied in clinical practice – for conditions such as ADHD, dementia, traumatic brain injury, and learning disorders – as well as in research, and is suitable for populations ranging from children to older adults, with specific norms by age group.

The BNT is one of the most widely used international instruments for assessing confrontational naming and lexical retrieval. It is based on the presentation of black-and-white drawings that participants must name, allowing the identification of language impairments frequently observed in aphasia, dementia, and other neurological conditions. Its applicability extends across children, adults, and older adults, and it is highly recognized in both clinical and research contexts. The test includes 60 line drawings presented in increasing order of difficulty, which must be named by the participant, identifying lexical retrieval deficits and anomia. Over the years, shorter versions of 15, 30, and 40 items have been developed, facilitating their use in different clinical and epidemiological contexts [61]. In Brazil, the BNT has been translated and adapted, with studies demonstrating strong educational influences on performance, a factor that must be considered when interpreting results [61]. Thus, the BNT remains a central tool for language and cognitive assessment in both clinical and research settings.

The Token Test, developed in Italy, was designed to identify subtle deficits in language comprehension in aphasic patients, particularly those not detected by routine clinical assessments. The test consists of oral commands involving the manipulation of tokens of different shapes, sizes, and colors, requiring patients to perform progressively more complex tasks [46]. Its main contribution lies in its ability to isolate linguistic processing difficulties while minimizing the influence of general intellectual factors. Initially aimed at adults with aphasia, the Token Test has since been widely used in both research and clinical contexts, becoming a sensitive tool for assessing verbal comprehension in diverse neurological populations. In Brazil, adaptation and standardization efforts have included a reduced version for older adults, which demonstrated good clinical applicability and relevance for national neuropsychology, helping address the scarcity of standardized tests in this context. The Token Test has therefore been consolidated internationally as a sensitive and reference tool for assessing verbal comprehension, with specific adaptations for the Brazilian setting [47].

The CANTAB, developed at the University of Cambridge, is a computerized battery designed for comprehensive cognitive evaluation. Initially applied to healthy older adults [48], it demonstrated sensitivity in detecting subtle cognitive changes and has since been widely used in clinical populations, including Alzheimer's disease, Parkinson's disease, schizophrenia, and mood disorders [49]. More recently, Cambridge Cognition has released web-based versions of the CANTAB, enabling remote or in-person administration in various clinical and research contexts. The digital platform retains the structure of the traditional subtests and provides automated reports covering domains such as attention, memory, executive functions, and processing speed, making it a scalable, standardized, and clinically useful tool for cognitive monitoring in diverse populations [62].

Given the wide range of instruments available, cognitive assessment is an indispensable resource for both clinical and scientific investigation of higher mental functions. The variety of tests – from brief screening measures to more complex and specific batteries – demonstrates that each tool has its own target population, applicability, and sensitivity, and must be selected according to the goals of the evaluation and the clinical context. Careful use of these instruments not only supports the early detection of cognitive alterations but also enables monitoring of clinical progression and the development of effective rehabilitation strategies, particularly in the context of an aging population.

4. Cognitive assessment in individuals with hearing loss

Cognitive assessment of individuals with hearing loss requires the use of instruments sensitive to the specificities of this population in order to minimize biases resulting from auditory alterations. If these particularities are not considered, test performance may be compromised, leading to misinterpretations of the individual's actual cognitive status. Accordingly, adapted versions of such instruments have been developed in recent decades, representing significant progress in cognitive screening for people with hearing impairment.

Among these initiatives are tools specifically designed for this population, such as the Montreal Cognitive Assessment – Hearing Impaired (MoCA-H) [63], the MoCA version for hearing aid users (MoCA-HA) [64], the Repeatable Battery for the Assessment of Neuropsychological Status – Hearing (RBANS-H) [65], and the computerized Auditory and Language-Independent Cognitive Test Battery (ALAcog) [66], which eliminate or minimize auditory stimuli in their instructions and tasks. These instruments represent important advances by enabling fairer and more reliable evaluations, reducing the influence of hearing on cognitive performance, and allowing for more accurate diagnoses and more appropriate clinical decision-making.

The MoCA-H was developed as an adaptation of the MoCA [36] to minimize bias caused by hearing loss during test administration. To achieve this, auditory-dependent items were replaced by visual and written stimuli, allowing individuals with hearing impairment to be more accurately evaluated across different cognitive domains [67]. The MoCA-H is intended for older adults aged 60 and over with moderate or more severe hearing loss, and it uses cards with written instructions to ensure comprehension of tasks. It assesses eight domains: executive functions, naming, attention, memory, abstract reasoning, orientation, delayed recall, visuospatial skills, and language [63]. Currently, several versions of the MoCA-H are available in different languages – including English, Arabic, Chinese, Dutch, German, Hungarian, Italian, Persian, Portuguese, and Spanish – expanding its international applicability across cultural and linguistic contexts [50]. Its validity and clinical applicability have been confirmed in multiple investigations. Initial studies already demonstrated satisfactory psychometric properties [67], and more recent validation reinforced its reliability in older populations with hearing loss [63]. In Brazil, the MoCA-H underwent cross-cultural adaptation in collaboration with the original authors and based on rigorous psychometric criteria [68]. Although available on the official website [50], normative data for the Brazilian population are not yet established, and ongoing studies aim to provide these benchmarks.

Another version, the MoCA-HA, was developed to assess cognition in older adults who use hearing aids. Adaptations were informed by health professionals – including psychiatrists, clinical psychologists, audiologists, hearing aid center managers, otolaryngologists, and vestibular physicians – as well as older adults with hearing impairment or dual sensory deficits (hearing and vision). The goal was to transform version 8.3 of the MoCA into a computer-based tool relying exclusively on visual input. This adaptation allows assessment regardless of the degree of hearing loss, while maintaining key cognitive domains such as attention, memory, language, and executive functions, and incorporating the Memory Index Score (MIS) subtask. Validation studies have shown high diagnostic accuracy in identifying cognitive impairment, although there are still fewer validation studies compared to the MoCA-H. Nonetheless, findings suggest that a visual approach, combined with expert feedback, provides more reliable and sensitive screening, reducing the impact of hearing loss on cognitive performance [64].

The RBANS [65] was originally developed as a brief cognitive battery for adults, covering five domains: immediate memory, delayed memory, attention, language, and visuospatial/constructional skills. To meet the needs of individuals with severe to profound hearing loss, particularly candidates for cochlear implantation, an adapted version (RBANS-H) was created. In this version, oral instructions and verbal stimuli in certain subtests (e.g., List Learning, Story Memory, Digit Span, and List Recognition) were supplemented with visual and written presentations, ensuring comprehension and avoiding the misinterpretation of hearing limitations as cognitive deficits. Maintaining the original structure and administration time (~30 minutes), the RBANS-H has been applied in longitudinal protocols, evaluating participants before and after cochlear implant activation. Some studies have reported improvements in memory and attention following auditory rehabilitation, suggesting that the battery is a feasible, sensitive, and reliable tool for monitoring cognitive changes in older adults with hearing impairment [69, 70, 71]. Thus, the RBANS-H has become a relevant tool for both clinical practice and research, providing fairer and more accurate evaluations of cognitive functions in individuals with hearing loss.

The ALAcog is a computerized neurocognitive battery developed in Germany to assess cognitive functions in individuals with hearing loss, particularly older adults and cochlear implant users. It consists of non-auditory and language-independent subtests, which significantly reduce biases from auditory processing and allow for a more accurate evaluation of cognitive performance in this population. The instrument has been applied in studies involving older adults with and without hearing loss, as well as cochlear implant patients, and has shown good clinical applicability [66, 72, 73]. Its structure evaluates multiple cognitive domains – including attention, short and long-term memory, working memory, executive functions, processing speed, and inhibition – using predominantly visual stimuli. The ALAcog, therefore, represents a sensitive, adapted, and promising tool for cognitive screening and monitoring in older adults and cochlear implant candidates or users, overcoming the limitations of traditional sound-based instruments [66].

Despite these advances in the development and adaptation of cognitive instruments for individuals with hearing loss, important limitations remain. Many available tests rely heavily on reading and written processing, which poses an additional barrier for populations with low literacy or limited educational backgrounds. This reliance can compromise validity, as performance may be more influenced by reading skills than by actual cognitive abilities. One study emphasized that the large proportion of older adults with low literacy or no formal education is at risk of misinterpretation when assessed with traditional tools, since these were largely developed around school-based tasks such as reading, writing, and arithmetic, potentially leading to inaccurate diagnoses of cognitive decline [74]. Furthermore, few instruments have been standardized on a large scale for populations with hearing loss, and there are still no tools specifically designed to comprehensively assess cognition in individuals with both hearing loss and low education levels. This underscores the need for continued research and innovation. In this context, the creation of truly inclusive tools – culturally adapted and independent of auditory or reading demands – represents a critical challenge to ensure fair and accurate cognitive assessment for this population.

5. Conclusion(s)

The high prevalence of hearing loss and its association with cognitive decline make it essential that cognitive assessment be conducted in an integrated, systematic manner that is sensitive to the specificities of this population. This involves reducing auditory pathway–related biases through visual or multimodal approaches, routinely including sensory screening in the diagnostic process, and interpreting results in light of sociodemographic variables, particularly education and age. Such precautions enhance diagnostic accuracy, guide more precise therapeutic strategies, and enable monitoring of clinical progression, supporting the preservation of communication, autonomy, and quality of life. Despite advances achieved, significant gaps remain in the assessment of individuals with low education levels, underscoring the need to develop truly inclusive instruments. In this context, interdisciplinary approaches – integrating auditory rehabilitation, cognitive stimulation strategies, and longitudinal follow-up – are fundamental to mitigating risks and promoting cognitive health throughout aging.

Acknowledgments

We thank the Research Support Foundation of the State of Rio Grande do Sul (FAPERGS) for the financial support provided through Grant Agreement nº 25/2551-0000857-3, which made this work possible.

Conflict of interest

The authors declare no conflict of interest.

Author details

Rochele Martins Machado*, Karina Carlesso Pagliarin and Fernanda Soares Aurélio Patatt
Federal University of Santa Maria, Santa Maria, Brazil

*Address all correspondence to: rochele.machado@acad.ufsm.br

References

[1] World Health Organization. World Report on Disability. Geneva: WHO; 2011

[2] World Health Organization. Deafness and hearing loss [Internet]. Geneva: World Health Organization; 2025 February 26. Available from: https://www.who.int/en/news-room/fact-sheets/detail/deafness-and-hearing-loss [Accessed: 2025-September-9]

[3] Kopper H, Teixeira AR, Dorneles S. Cognitive performance of a group of elders: Influence of hearing, age, sex, and education. Archives of Otorhinolaryngology. 2009;**13**:39–43. https://arquivosdeorl.org.br/conteudo/acervo_eng.asp?Id=586

[4] Golub JS, Brickman AM, Ciarleglio AJ, Schupf N, Luchsinger JA. Association of subclinical hearing loss with cognitive performance. JAMA Otolaryngology–Head & Neck Surgery. 2020;**146**(1):57–67. DOI: 10.1001/jamaoto.2019.3375

[5] Lin FR, Metter EJ, O'Brien RJ, Resnick SM, Zonderman AB, Ferrucci L. Hearing loss and incident dementia. Archives of Neurology. 2011;**68**(2):214–220. DOI: 10.1001/archneurol.2010.362

[6] Lin FR, Yaffe K, Xia J, Xue QL, Harris TB, Purchase-Helzner E, et al. Hearing loss and cognitive decline in older adults. JAMA Internal Medicine. 2013;**173**(4):293–299. DOI: 10.1001/jamainternmed.2013.1868

[7] Loughrey DG, Kelly ME, Kelley GA, Brennan S, Lawlor BA. Association of age-related hearing loss with cognitive function, cognitive impairment, and dementia: A systematic review and meta-analysis. JAMA Otolaryngology–Head & Neck Surgery. 2018;**144**(2):115–126. DOI: 10.1001/jamaoto.2017.2513

[8] Livingston G, Huntley J, Sommerlad A, Ames D, Ballard C, Banerjee S, et al. Dementia prevention, intervention, and care: 2020 report of the Lancet Commission. The Lancet. 2020;**396**(10248):413–446. DOI: 10.1001/jamaoto.2019.3375

[9] Fulton SE, Lister JJ, Bush AL, Edwards JD, Andel R. Mechanisms of the hearing-cognition relationship. Seminars in Hearing. 2015;**36**(3):140–149. DOI: 10.1055/s-0035-1555117

[10] Sharma A, Glick H. Cross-modal re-organization in clinical populations with hearing loss. Brain Sciences. 2016;**6**(1):4. DOI: 10.1001/jamainternmed.2013.1868

[11] Pichora-Fuller MK, Mick P, Reed M. Hearing, cognition, and healthy aging: Social and public health implications of the links between age-related declines in hearing and cognition. Seminars in Hearing. 2015;**36**(3):122–139. DOI: 10.1001/jamaoto.2017.2513

[12] Borges MGS, Santos Penna LM, Lessa AH, Jotz GP, Soldera CLC, Machado MS. Correlações entre a avaliação audiológica e a triagem cognitiva em idosos. Revista CEFAC. 2016;**18**(6):1285–1293. DOI: 10.1590/1982-021620161865616

[13] Ren F, Ma W, Li M, Sun H, Xin Q, Zong W, et al. Hearing loss and cognition among older adults in a Han Chinese cohort. Frontiers in Neuroscience. 2019;**13**:632

[14] Füllgrabe C. Auditory biases in cognitive assessment: Insights from a hearing-loss simulation for the screening of dementia due to Alzheimer's disease. Journal of Alzheimer's Disease. 2023;**91**(2): 537–541. DOI: 10.3233/JAD-215695

[15] Ferguson MA, Nakano K, Jayakody DMP. Clinical assessment tools for the detection of cognitive impairment and hearing loss in the ageing population: A scoping review. Clinical Interventions in Aging. 2023;**18**:2041–2051. DOI: 10.2147/CIA.S409114

[16] Slade K, Plack CJ, Nuttall HE. The effects of age-related hearing loss on the brain and cognitive function. Trends in Neurosciences. 2020;**43**(10):810–821. DOI: 10.1016/j.tins.2020.07.005

[17] Livingston G, Huntley J, Sommerlad A, Ames D, Ballard C, Banerjee S, et al. Dementia prevention, intervention, and care: 2024 report of the Lancet Commission. Lancet. 2024;**404**(10452):572–628. DOI: 10.1016/S0140-6736(24)01296-0

[18] Tomida K, Shimoda T, Nakajima C, Kawakami A, Shimada H. Risk of dementia with hearing impairment and social isolation. Alzheimer's & Dementia: Diagnosis, Assessment & Disease Monitoring. 2024;**16**(2):e12586. DOI: 10.1002/dad2.12586

[19] Wu F, Zhou C. Hearing loss and cognitive function: Mediating role of social isolation and depression. American Journal of Alzheimer's Disease & Other Dementias. 2024;**39**:15333175241227318. DOI: 10.1177/15333175241227318

[20] Agência USP. Perda auditiva é associada a declínio cognitivo mais acelerado, confirma estudo com brasileiros. [Internet]. São Paulo: Jornal USP; 2025 February 26. Available from: https://jornal.usp.br/ciencias/ciencias-da-saude/perda-auditiva-e-associada-a-declinio-cognitivo-mais-acelerado-confirma-estudo-com-brasileiros/ [Accessed: 2025-September-7]

[21] Myrstad C, Engdahl BL, Costafreda SG, Krokstad S, Lin F, Livingston G, et al. Hearing impairment and risk of dementia in the HUNT study (HUNT4 70+): A Norwegian cohort study. EClinicalMedicine. 2023;**66**:102319. DOI: 10.1016/j.eclinm.2023.102319

[22] Chen Y, Wong LLN, Chan SS, Yu J. Speech perception in noise is associated with different cognitive abilities in Chinese-speaking older adults with and without hearing aids. Frontiers in Psychology. 2022;**12**:640300. DOI: 10.3389/fpsyg.2021.640300

[23] Uchida Y, Sugiura S, Nishita Y, Saji N, Sone M, Ueda H. Age-related hearing loss and cognitive decline: The potential mechanisms linking the two. Auris Nasus Larynx. 2019;**46**(1):1–9. DOI: 10.1016/j.anl.2018.08.010

[24] Samelli AG, Gonçalves NG, Fyomm P, Guesser VM, Matas CG, Rabelo CM, et al. Hearing loss and cognitive decline in the Brazilian Longitudinal Study of Adult Health (ELSA-Brasil) during eight years of follow-up. Journal of Alzheimer's Disease. 2025;**104**(1):283–293. DOI: 10.1177/13872877251315043

[25] Liu K. Hearing intervention and cognitive decline: The ACHIEVE trial. The Lancet. 2024;**404**(10447):29–30. DOI: 10.1016/S0140-6736(24)00712-8

[26] Cantuaria ML, Pedersen ER, Waldorff FB, et al. Hearing loss, hearing aid use, and risk of dementia in older adults. JAMA Otolaryngology–Head & Neck Surgery. 2024;**150**(2):157–164. DOI: 10.1001/jamaoto.2023.3509

[27] Qian ZJ, Wattamwar K, Caruana FF, Otter J, Leskowitz MJ, Siedlecki B, Spitzer JB, Lalwani AK. Hearing Aid Use is Associated with Better Mini-Mental State Exam Performance. The American Journal of Geriatric Psychiatry. 2016;**24** (9):694–702. DOI: 10.1016/j.jagp.2016.03.005

[28] Bucholc M, Schembri A, Busby P, et al. The impact of hearing impairment and hearing aid use on cognitive function in older adults: A longitudinal study. Alzheimer's & Dementia: Translational Research & Clinical Interventions. 2022;**8**(1):e12248. DOI: 10.1002/trc2.12248

[29] Sarant JZ, Busby PA, Schembri A, et al. A hearing aid could extend your brain function by years. Pursuit. 2024 Disponível em: https://pursuit.unimelb.edu.au/articles/a-hearing-aid-could-extend-your-brain-function-by-years [Accessed: 2025-September-15]

[30] Lezak MD, Howieson DB, Bigler ED, Tranel D. Neuropsychological Assessment. 5th ed. New York: Oxford University Press; 2012

[31] Carone DAS, E SEMS, Spreen O. A compendium of neuropsychological tests: Administration, norms, and commentary. 3rd ed. New York: Oxford University Press; 2006. Revista de Neuropsicologia Aplicada. 2007;**14** (1):62–63. DOI: 10.1080/09084280701280502

[32] Petersen RC, Lopez O, Armstrong MJ, Getchius TSD, Ganguli M, Gloss D, et al. Practice guideline update summary: Mild cognitive impairment. Report of the guideline development, dissemination, and implementation subcommittee of the American Academy of Neurology. Neurology. 2018;**90**(3):126–135. DOI: 10.1212/WNL.0000000000004826

[33] Gauthier S, Reisberg B, Zaudig M, Petersen RC, Ritchie K, Broich K, et al. Mild cognitive impairment. Lancet. 2006;**367** (9518):1262–1270. DOI: 10.1016/S0140-6736(06)68542-5

[34] Albert MS, DeKosky ST, Dickson D, Dubois B, Feldman HH, Fox NC, et al. The diagnosis of mild cognitive impairment due to Alzheimer's disease: Recommendations from the National Institute on Aging-Alzheimer's Association workgroups. Alzheimer's & Dementia. 2011;**7** (3):270–279. DOI: 10.1016/j.jalz.2011.03.008

[35] Folstein MF, Folstein SE, McHugh PR. "Mini-mental state". A practical method for grading the cognitive state of patients for the clinician. Journal of Psychiatric Research. 1975;**12**(3):189–198. DOI: 10.1016/0022-3956(75)90026-6

[36] Nasreddine ZS, Phillips NA, Bédirian V, Charbonneau S, Whitehead V, Collin I, et al. The Montreal Cognitive Assessment, MoCA: A brief screening tool for mild cognitive impairment. Journal of the American Geriatrics Society. 2005;**53** (4):695–699. DOI: 10.1111/j.1532-5415.2005.53221.x

[37] Rosen WG, Mohs RC, Davis KL. A new rating scale for Alzheimer's disease. American Journal of Psychiatry.

1984;**141**(11):1356–1364. DOI: 10.1176/ajp.141.11.1356

[38] Dubois B, Slachevsky A, Litvan I, Pillon B. The FAB: A frontal assessment battery at bedside. Neurology. 2000;**55**(11):1621–1626. DOI: 10.1212/wnl.55.11.1621

[39] Stroop JR. Studies of interference in serial verbal reactions. Journal of Experimental Psychology. 1935;**18**(6):643–662. DOI: 10.1037/h0054651

[40] Grant DA, Berg EA. A behavioral analysis of degree of reinforcement and ease of shifting to new responses in a Weigl-type card-sorting problem. Journal of Experimental Psychology. 1948;**38**(4):404–411. DOI: 10.1037/h0059831

[41] Rey A. L'Examen Clinique En Psychologie. Paris: Press Universitaire de France; 1958

[42] Wechsler D. A standardized memory scale for clinical use. The Journal of Psychology. 1945;**19**(1):87–95. DOI: 10.1080/00223980.1945.9917223

[43] Reitan RM. Validity of the Trail Making Test as an indicator of organic brain damage. Perceptual and Motor Skills. 1958;**8**(3):271–276. DOI: 10.2466/pms.1958.8.3.271

[44] Wechsler D. Manual for the Wechsler Intelligence Scale for Children-Revised. New York: Harcourt Test Publishers; 1997

[45] Kaplan E, Goodglass H, Weintraub S. The Boston Naming Test. Philadelphia: Lea & Febiger; 1983

[46] De Renzi E, Vignolo LA. The token test: A sensitive test to detect receptive disturbances in aphasics. Brain. 1962;**85**(4):665–678. DOI: 10.1093/brain/85.4.665

[47] Moreira L, Schlottfeldt CG, Paula JJ, Daniel MT, Paiva A, Cazita V, et al. Estudo normativo do Token Test versão reduzida: Dados preliminares para uma população de idosos brasileiros. Archives of Clinical Psychiatry (São Paulo). 2011;**38**(3):97–101. DOI: 10.1590/S0101-60832011000300003

[48] Robbins TW, James M, Owen AM, Sahakian BJ, McInnes L, Rabbitt P. Cambridge Neuropsychological Test Automated Battery (CANTAB): A factor analytic study of a large sample of normal elderly volunteers. Dementia. 1994;**5**(5):266–281. DOI: 10.1159/000106735

[49] Sahakian BJ, Owen AM. Computerized assessment in neuropsychiatry using CANTAB: Discussion paper. Journal of the Royal Society of Medicine. 1992;**85**(7):399–402

[50] MoCA Cognition. Papers [Internet]. Montreal: MoCA Cognition; Available from: https://mocacognition.com/paper/ [Accessed: 2025-September-16]

[51] Memória CM, Yassuda MS, Nakano EY, Forlenza OV. Brief screening for mild cognitive impairment: Validation of the Brazilian version of the Montreal cognitive assessment. International Journal of Geriatric Psychiatry. 2013;**28**(1):34–40. DOI: 10.1002/gps.3787

[52] Cecato JF, Montiel JM, Bartholomeu D, Martinelli JE. Poder preditivo do MoCA na avaliação neuropsicológica de pacientes com

diagnóstico de demência. Revista Brasileira de Geriatria E Gerontologia. 2014;**17**(4):707–719. DOI: 10.1590/1809-9823.2014.13123

[53] Cesar KG, Yassuda MS, Porto FHG, Brucki SMD, Nitrini R. MoCA test: Normative and diagnostic accuracy data for seniors with heterogeneous educational level in Brazil. Arquivos de Neuro-Psiquiatria. 2019;**77**(11):775–781. DOI: 10.1590/0004-282X20190130

[54] Beato RG. Versão brasileira da Bateria de Avaliação Frontal (FAB). Dementia & Neuropsychologia. 2007;**1**(4):201–207. DOI: 10.1590/S1980-57642008DN10400006

[55] Malloy-Diniz LF, Lasmar VAP, Gazinelli LSR, Fuentes D, Salgado JV. The Rey Auditory-Verbal Learning Test: Applicability for the Brazilian elderly population. Revista Brasileira de Psiquiatria. 2007;**29**(4):324–329. DOI: 10.1590/S1516-44462006005000053

[56] Cotta MF, Malloy-Diniz LF, Fuentes D, Nicolato R, Moraes EN, Miranda DM. O teste de aprendizagem auditivo-verbal de Rey (RAVLT) no diagnóstico diferencial do envelhecimento cognitivo normal e patológico. Contextos Clínicos. 2012;**5**(1):10–25. DOI: 10.4013/ctc.2012.51.02

[57] Ferman TJ, Smith GE, Boeve BF, Ivnik RJ, Petersen RC, Knopman D, et al. Neuropsychological differentiation of dementia with Lewy bodies from normal aging and Alzheimer's disease. Clinical Neuropsychologist. 2005;**19**(1):107–121. DOI: 10.1080/13854040490507189

[58] Dzikon C. The Wechsler Memory Scale (WMS-IV). In Carducci BJ, Nave CS, editors. The Wiley Encyclopedia of Personality and Individual Differences: Measurement and Assessment. 1st ed. Hoboken (NJ): John Wiley & Sons; 2020. 529–532 p. DOI: 10.1002/9781119547167.ch159

[59] Campanholo KR, Romão MA, Machado MAR, Serrao VT, Coutinho DGC, Benute GRG, et al. Performance of an adult Brazilian sample on the Trail Making Test and Stroop Test. Dementia & Neuropsychologia. 2014;**8**(1):26–31. DOI: 10.1590/S1980-57642014DN81000005

[60] Iuculano T, Moro R, Butterworth B. Updating working memory and arithmetical attainment in school. Learning and Individual Differences. 2011;**21**(6):655–661. DOI: 10.1016/j.lindif.2010.12.002

[61] Miotto EC, Sato J, Lucia MCS, Camargo CHP, Scaff M. Development of an adapted version of the Boston Naming Test for Portuguese speakers. Revista Brasileira de Psiquiatria. 2010;**32**(3):279–282. DOI: 10.1590/S1516-44462010005000006

[62] Cambridge Cognition. CANTAB®: Completed Web Test [Internet]. 2025. Available from: https://cambridgecognition.com/completed-web-test/ [Accessed: 2025-February-20]

[63] Dawes P, Reeves D, Yeung WK, Holland F, Charalambous AP, Côté M, et al. Development and validation of the Montreal cognitive assessment for people with hearing impairment (MoCA-H). Journal of the American Geriatrics Society. 2023;**71**(5):1485–1494. DOI: 10.1111/jgs.18241

[64] Utoomprurkporn N, Stott J, Costafreda SG, North C, Heatley M, Bamiou DE. The screening accuracy of a visually based Montreal Cognitive

Assessment tool for older adult hearing aid users. Frontiers in Aging Neuroscience. 2021;**13**:706282. DOI: 10.3389/fnagi.2021.706282

[65] Randolph C, Tierney MC, Mohr E, Chase TN. The Repeatable Battery for the Assessment of Neuropsychological Status (RBANS): Preliminary clinical validity. Journal of Clinical and Experimental Neuropsychology. 1998;**20**(3):310–319. DOI: 10.1076/jcen.20.3.310.823

[66] Völter C, Götze L, Falkenstein M, Dazert S, Thomas JP. Application of a computer-based neurocognitive assessment battery in the elderly with and without hearing loss. Clinical Interventions in Aging. 2017;**12**:1681–1690. DOI: 10.2147/CIA.S142541

[67] Lin VYW, Chung J, Callahan BL, Smith L, Gritters N, Chen JM, et al. Development of cognitive screening test for the severely hearing impaired: Hearing-impaired MoCA. Laryngoscope. 2017;**127**(Suppl 1):S4–11. DOI: 10.1002/lary.26590

[68] Machado RM, Pagliarin KC, Patatt FSA. Montreal Cognitive Assessment Hearing Impairment (MoCA-H): Cross-cultural adaptation to Brazilian Portuguese. CoDAS. 2025;**37**(1):e20240125. Available from: DOI: 10.1590/2317-1782/e20240125en

[69] Claes AJ, Mertens G, Gilles A, Hofkens-van den Brandt A, Fransen E, Van Rompaey V, et al. The Repeatable Battery for the Assessment of Neuropsychological Status for Hearing Impaired Individuals (RBANS-H) before and after cochlear implantation: A protocol for a prospective, longitudinal cohort study. Frontiers in Neuroscience. 2016;**10**:512. PMID: 27895549. DOI: 10.3389/fnins.2016.00512

[70] Gommeren H, Vandenbroeke T, Bosmans J, Mertens G, Cras P, Engelborghs S, Van Ombergen A, Gilles A, Lammers M, Van Rompaey V. Sensorineural hearing loss negatively impacts cognition in older subjects with normal lateral semi-circular canal function. Audiology and Neuro-Otology. 2025;**30**(2):109–117. Epub 2024 Oct 22. PMID:39437745. DOI: 10.1159/000541436

[71] Vandenbroeke T, Andries E, Lammers MJ, Van de Heyning P, Hofkens-van den Brandt A, Vanderveken O, Van Rompaey V, Mertens G. Alterações cognitivas até 4 anos após implante coclear em idosos: Um estudo longitudinal prospectivo usando o RBANS-H. Ear and Hearing. 2025;**46**(2):361–370. DOI: 10.1097/AUD.0000000000001583

[72] Hamerschmidt R, Santos VM, Gonçalves FM, Delcenserie A, Champoux F, de Araujo CM, de Lacerda ABM. Cognitive performance changes after cochlear implantation in adults and elderly: A systematic review and meta-analysis. International Journal of Audiology. 2022;**62**(6):521–532. DOI: 10.1080/14992027.2022.2050823

[73] Götze L, Sheikh F, Haubitz I, Falkenstein M, Timmesfeld N, Völter C. Evaluation of a non-auditory neurocognitive test battery in hearing-impaired according to age. European Archives of Oto-Rhino-Laryngology. 2024;**281**(6):2941–2949. Epub 2024 Jan 9. PMID:38191747. DOI: 10.1007/s00405-023-08408-9

[74] Kosmidis MH. Challenges in the neuropsychological assessment of illiterate older adults. Language, Cognition and Neuroscience. 2017;**33**(3):373–386. DOI: 10.1080/23273798.2017.1379605

Section 4

Treatment and Rehabilitation

Chapter 5

Perspective Chapter: Neuromodulation in Tinnitus – Recent Advances and Therapeutic Perspectives

Thiago Silva Almeida de Souza and Lisiane Holdefer

Abstract

Neuromodulation has emerged as an innovative and essential therapeutic alternative for the management of tinnitus, particularly in patients who are refractory to conventional treatment approaches. Tinnitus is a complex and multifactorial condition, often associated with maladaptive neuroplastic changes within auditory and non-auditory neural networks, which contributes to symptom persistence and functional impairment. In this context, neuromodulation techniques aim to directly influence dysfunctional neural activity involved in tinnitus generation and maintenance. Among the most studied approaches are transcranial direct current stimulation (tDCS), transcutaneous vagus nerve stimulation (tVNS), transcranial alternating current stimulation (tACS), and photobiomodulation. These modalities target cortical and subcortical circuits related to auditory perception, attention, and emotional processing. Recent evidence suggests that when applied individually or in combined therapeutic protocols, these techniques may lead to significant reductions in tinnitus intensity, perceptual awareness, and associated distress. Consequently, improvements in quality of life and functional outcomes have been reported in different clinical populations. In addition, neuromodulation techniques generally demonstrate a favorable safety profile, with a low incidence of mild and transient adverse effects, reinforcing their clinical feasibility. In a therapeutic landscape characterized by limited treatment options and heterogeneous clinical responses, neuromodulation represents a promising and expanding field. However, despite encouraging results, important challenges remain. There is a clear need for robust, well-designed clinical trials to standardize stimulation parameters, define optimal treatment protocols, and identify patient-specific predictors of response. Considering the substantial functional, emotional, and social impact of tinnitus, the advancement and refinement of neuromodulation-based interventions constitute both a scientific priority and a clinical imperative.

Keywords: tinnitus, neuromodulation, transcranial direct current stimulation (tDCS), transcranial magnetic stimulation (rTMS), photobiomodulation

1. Introduction

Tinnitus affects approximately 14.4% of the global population, equivalent to 740 million adults, of whom around 120 million experience severe forms. Its prevalence varies across continents due to epidemiological, environmental, and methodological factors. In Asia, the average prevalence is 15.2%, close to the global rate, although internal variability is substantial: in South Korea, about 20% of the population reports tinnitus, often associated with older age, depression, and noise exposure [1]. In China, studies indicate prevalence ranging from 4.3% to 51.3%, with higher rates observed among the elderly [2]. In South America, population-based studies report prevalence as high as 21.9%, possibly linked to greater occupational noise exposure and low adherence to hearing protection use [1]. In North America and Europe, prevalence rates are around 14%, with a greater impact on older adults and individuals with chronic conditions [1]. In Africa, data remain scarce and are limited by underdiagnosis and methodological weaknesses [1], while in Oceania, prevalence is estimated at 15%, often associated with hearing loss and noise exposure [1].

From a neurofunctional perspective, tinnitus extends beyond the peripheral auditory system. Alterations in the salience network (SN), default mode network (DMN), and central executive network (CEN) contribute to the intrusive perception of the symptom and its emotional impact [3, 4]. The SN assigns relevance to the sound, the DMN integrates it into internal experience, and the CEN fails to redirect attention, sustaining a cycle of distress. This process is further reinforced by neurochemical imbalances, such as elevated glutamate and reduced GABA levels, which promote neuronal hyperexcitability [5]. Additionally, decreased levels of brain-derived neurotrophic factor (BDNF) in auditory and limbic regions are associated with greater tinnitus intensity and chronic stress [6]. Complementary models include stochastic resonance, where the brain amplifies neural noise to compensate for hearing loss, and predictive coding, which explains symptom persistence as a failure to correct prediction errors [7].

Clinically, tinnitus poses significant challenges due to its subjective nature and complex neurophysiology. Despite advances in sound therapies, auditory rehabilitation, and counseling, many patients with moderate to severe presentations show inadequate responses, often due to the lack of standardized protocols and the difficulty in objectively measuring treatment outcomes [1, 8]. In this context, interest in neuromodulation has grown. This technique aims to modulate cortical excitability and connectivity, representing a promising alternative for tinnitus management [1, 8].

2. Physiological and neurobiological bases of tinnitus

Tinnitus may originate in the cochlea, through cervicogenic somatosensory mechanisms, or from central processes. Cochlear alterations, such as outer hair cell dysfunction and synaptopathy, reduce auditory input even in individuals with normal audiometric thresholds. These changes may result from noise exposure, aging, or ototoxicity and can lead to incoherent spontaneous firing of the auditory nerve, triggering compensatory responses within the central nervous system (CNS) [9]. Following hearing loss, cortical reorganization occurs in the primary auditory cortex, marked by neural hyperactivity and desynchronization. The secondary and lateral auditory cortices contribute to tinnitus perception by influencing its localization and perceptual content. Cortical expansion of the affected frequency regions enhances internal perception and promotes symptom chronification [9].

Tinnitus may also be modulated by cervical (C2–C8) and trigeminal nerve afferents, which are integrated into the dorsal cochlear nucleus. This integration can produce synaptic reorganization and neural activity patterns similar to those found in cochlear tinnitus [9]. Overall, the loss of afferent stimuli alters neuroplasticity in central auditory pathways, inducing hyperactivity and desynchronization in structures such as the dorsal cochlear nucleus, medial geniculate body, inferior colliculus, and primary auditory cortex. These changes reflect maladaptive neuroplasticity, whereby the brain interprets the absence of external stimuli as a phantom sound [9].

2.1 Limbic system

The consolidation of memories and emotional responses associated with tinnitus involves central components of the limbic system, such as the amygdala and hippocampus, both located in the temporal lobe. The amygdala plays a key role in processing emotions such as fear and anxiety. It contributes to the formation of emotional memory and modulates the hypothalamic-pituitary-adrenal (HPA) axis response related to stress. The hippocampus, in turn, is essential for the creation of new declarative memories, the consolidation of short-term into long-term experiences, and the spatial and contextual mapping of events. It also regulates emotional aspects and interacts with the amygdala in affective responses [10].

In the context of tinnitus, the amygdala assigns a negative emotional valence to the perception, such as threat and discomfort. When persistently activated, it intensifies stress, anxiety, and emotional suffering. The hippocampus contributes to the encoding and consolidation of tinnitus-related memory, enabling the perception of sound even in the absence of peripheral auditory stimuli through the reconsolidation of neural patterns [10].

Together, these two structures form a negative reinforcement circuit: tinnitus, once perceived, is associated with negative emotions, becomes fixed in memory, and is perpetuated by emotional activation, which hinders attentional redirection.

2.2 Dorsolateral prefrontal cortex (dlpfc)

The dorsolateral prefrontal cortex (DLPFC) plays a crucial role in executive functions and emotional regulation. Its activation promotes top-down modulation of the amygdala, thereby reducing the affective load of tinnitus and facilitating the cognitive reappraisal of negative memories. In situations of heightened anxiety or stress, bottom-up modulation occurs, in which the amygdala influences the DLPFC and exacerbates tinnitus perception. Furthermore, the DLPFC indirectly affects the hippocampus through executive–limbic networks, modulating the emotional consolidation of tinnitus [10].

2.3 Anterior cingulate cortex (acc)

The anterior cingulate cortex (ACC), subdivided into dorsal (dACC) and rostral (rACC) regions, assigns emotional significance to tinnitus and plays a key role in the neural noise-canceling function, which filters out irrelevant auditory signals. Dysfunctions of the rACC are associated with the persistent perception of tinnitus, with functional magnetic resonance imaging studies revealing alterations in this region among chronic patients. Neurochemical changes in the ACC may also contribute to the persistence of the symptom [11].

2.4 Attention and resting-state networks

In chronic tinnitus, there is a functional reorganization of major brain networks, particularly the default mode network (DMN) and the salience network, which helps explain its persistence and profound emotional impact.

2.4.1 Default mode network (dmn)

The default mode network (DMN) comprises a set of brain regions that exhibit increased activation during mental rest states, when the individual is not engaged in external tasks. In patients with chronic tinnitus, studies have shown that this network integrates the tinnitus sound into automatic mental activities, a phenomenon described as *embedding* or *embodiment* [3, 4]. As a result, even during rest, the brain continues to process tinnitus as part of the individual's internal experience or identity, making suppression more difficult. This integration sustains constant attentional focus on the sound and amplifies emotional distress by signaling to the brain that the stimulus holds high salience. Evidence of this mechanism is seen in the increased functional connectivity between the DMN, auditory structures, and limbic regions [3, 4].

2.4.2 Salience network (sn)

The salience network (SN), located in the insula and dorsal anterior cingulate cortex, is responsible for detecting relevant stimuli and coordinating the transition between the default mode network (DMN) and the central executive network (CEN). In patients with chronic tinnitus, functional alterations in this network heighten the perception of sound and hinder attentional disengagement, thereby intensifying discomfort and impairing executive functions [3, 4].

The Triple Network Model describes the dysfunctional interaction between the DMN, SN, and CEN in tinnitus: the DMN integrates the sound into internal experience, the SN tags it as salient, and the CEN fails to redirect attention, creating a cycle of intrusive attention and emotional distress [3].

From a neurochemical perspective, the imbalance between excitatory and inhibitory neurotransmitters, such as glutamate and GABA, contributes to neuronal hyperexcitability in central auditory pathways, supporting the persistence of tinnitus [5]. Brain-derived neurotrophic factor (BDNF) also plays a key role in synaptic plasticity; reduced BDNF levels in auditory and limbic regions have been associated with greater tinnitus intensity and emotional alterations, suggesting a correlation with prolonged stress [6].

Complementary computational models include the stochastic resonance theory, in which the brain amplifies neural noise to compensate for reduced auditory input, and predictive coding theory, which posits that tinnitus arises from a failure to correct prediction errors [7].

3. Clinical classifications of tinnitus

3.1 Subjective and objective tinnitus

Tinnitus can be classified as either subjective or objective. The vast majority of patients, approximately 99%, report perceiving tinnitus without any externally detectable sound source; in such cases, it is classified as subjective tinnitus, typically associated with alterations in the auditory or central nervous system [8]. In contrast, objective tinnitus is rare, accounting for less than 1% of cases, and can be perceived through medical evaluation. It is often caused by physical factors such as vascular anomalies or muscular contractions in the ear region [8]. This distinction is essential for both diagnostic assessment and therapeutic management.

3.2 Pathophysiological classification of tinnitus

Although tinnitus may arise from multiple mechanisms, the most common types include cochlear, somatosensory, and psychogenic tinnitus.

3.2.1 Tinnitus cochlear

Cochlear tinnitus is frequently associated with damage to outer hair cells, synaptopathy, cochlear neurodegeneration, or ototoxicity. These conditions reduce sensory input and trigger central compensatory mechanisms. This process generates spontaneous and synchronized neural activity in the auditory system, which is perceived as tinnitus [9]. Some individuals with tinnitus present normal results on conventional audiometry, supporting the hypothesis that hidden cochlear damage, such as synaptopathy, may initiate the central hyperactivity linked to the symptom [9]. Research indicates that, following cochlear injury, reorganization occurs within the central auditory system, particularly in the dorsal cochlear nucleus and auditory cortex, allowing tinnitus to persist even after the peripheral lesion has stabilized.

3.2.2 Somatosensory tinnitus

Somatosensory or cervicogenic tinnitus is triggered by manipulations of the neck, jaw, eyes, or cervical muscle fibers. Patients typically do not present with hearing loss. In such cases, communication occurs between the somatosensory system (trigeminal nerve, cervical ganglia C2–C8) and the auditory system, primarily the dorsal cochlear nucleus (DCN). This mechanism increases neural excitability and results in the perception of tinnitus, affecting both its intensity and frequency [12].

3.2.3 Psychogenic tinnitus

Psychogenic tinnitus is associated with emotional and psychiatric factors. Individuals with this condition often do not exhibit peripheral auditory alterations. Mood disturbances, stress, anxiety, and sleep disorders influence both the perception of tinnitus and the level of distress it causes. When the symptom is linked to depression, anxiety, or sleep impairment, it may take on a catastrophic character, making it more difficult for the individual to adapt [13]. Additionally, emotional factors related to tinnitus may involve changes in executive functions and mild impairments in tasks requiring attentional control or working memory, thereby amplifying complaints related to the symptom [13].

4. Current therapeutic approaches and their limitations

Currently, various therapeutic approaches are employed in the management of tinnitus, including auditory rehabilitation in cases of hearing loss, sound therapy, counseling, lifestyle modifications, and, in some cases, pharmacological interventions. Each of these strategies demonstrates a certain degree of efficacy but also presents important limitations that hinder treatment success, especially in more severe or chronic cases.

- **Auditory rehabilitation and use of hearing aids (HA):** The use of hearing aids in patients with both hearing loss and tinnitus is important for restoring auditory input. They help prevent sensory deprivation and enhance neuroplasticity in the central auditory system, contributing to a reduction in tinnitus perception [8].

- **Sound therapy:** This involves the use of specific sound stimuli, which can be tailored based on the type and frequency of the tinnitus [8].

- **Auditory training:** Composed of active auditory exercises, this approach helps improve tinnitus perception, particularly in cases that show residual inhibition during masking tests [12].

- **Pharmacological treatment:** Some antidepressants, anticonvulsants, and anxiolytics are used, though there is strong evidence indicating limited efficacy.

- **Counseling and cognitive behavioral therapy (CBT):** These focus on stress management and tinnitus perception. They have shown the ability to reduce the emotional distress associated with the symptom, promoting improved quality of life and habituation [8, 11].

5. Neuromodulation

Neuromodulation comprises therapeutic techniques aimed at modifying neuronal activity by adjusting excitability, synchronization, and synaptic plasticity. These mechanisms result in electrical, chemical, and physiological changes that influence neuroplasticity. The goal is to target specific neural networks, promoting functional reorganization or controlling dysfunctional circuits associated with the symptoms [14]. The mode of action of neuromodulation depends on the technique employed, which can be invasive (such as vagus nerve stimulation or deep brain stimulation) or noninvasive (such as repetitive transcranial magnetic stimulation, transcranial direct current stimulation, transcranial alternating current stimulation, and low-level photobiomodulation) [15].

5.1 Types of neuromodulations: General concepts

5.1.1 Repetitive transcranial magnetic stimulation (rtms)

Repetitive transcranial magnetic stimulation (rTMS) is a noninvasive technique that uses magnetic fields to modulate cortical excitability. It involves the application of repetitive magnetic pulses to specific regions of the brain, typically the auditory cortex or the dorsolateral prefrontal cortex, depending on the therapeutic objective. Low-frequency rTMS (usually 1 Hz) is used to inhibit cortical hyperactivity, whereas high-frequency stimulation (>5 Hz) tends to facilitate excitatory responses (**Table 1**).

In tinnitus treatment, rTMS aims to reduce the hyperactivity and abnormal synchrony observed in the auditory cortex and related networks. Several clinical trials have demonstrated its potential to attenuate tinnitus intensity and associated distress, especially in chronic cases (**Table 1**). However, the results are heterogeneous and depend on factors such as coil positioning, stimulation parameters, session duration, and individual neurophysiological characteristics [16–18].

5.1.2 Transcranial direct current stimulation (tdcs)

tDCS is a noninvasive neuromodulation technique that uses a low-intensity electrical current, typically not exceeding 2 mA, applied through rubber electrodes covered with saline-soaked sponges placed on the scalp, aiming to alter the brain's electrical activity in the targeted region (**Figure 1**). This type of stimulation does not directly trigger neuronal firing but subtly modulates the membrane potential of neurons, facilitating or inhibiting their excitability [23].

Two types of electrodes are used in tDCS: the positive electrode (anode), which facilitates neural excitability, and the negative electrode (cathode), which

Author/Year [Ref]	Sample/Study type	Protocol	Main findings
Khedr et al., 2008 [17]	66 patients; RCT	1 Hz, temporoparietal cortex; 10 sessions	Significant reduction in loudness and distress vs. sham; effect partially maintained at follow-up
Khedr et al., 2010 [18]	80 patients; RCT	1 Hz ipsilateral vs. contralateral; 10 sessions	Greater benefit with ipsilateral low-frequency stimulation; significant clinical improvement
Plewnia et al., 2012 [19]	48 patients; RCT (3 arms)	Bilateral theta-burst (cTBS); 20 sessions	Active group showed significant clinical improvement
Folmer et al., 2015 [20]	64 patients; RCT	Left DLPFC, 10 Hz; 10 sessions	Significant improvement in TFI/THI sustained up to 26 weeks
Landgrebe et al., 2017 [21]	146 patients; multicenter RCT	1 Hz, left temporal lobe; 10 sessions	No significant difference vs. sham; high response variability
Liang et al., 2020 [22]	Meta-analysis; 20 studies	Various targets and protocols	Confirms efficacy, but highlights need for

Table 1.
Studies on rTMS in tinnitus.

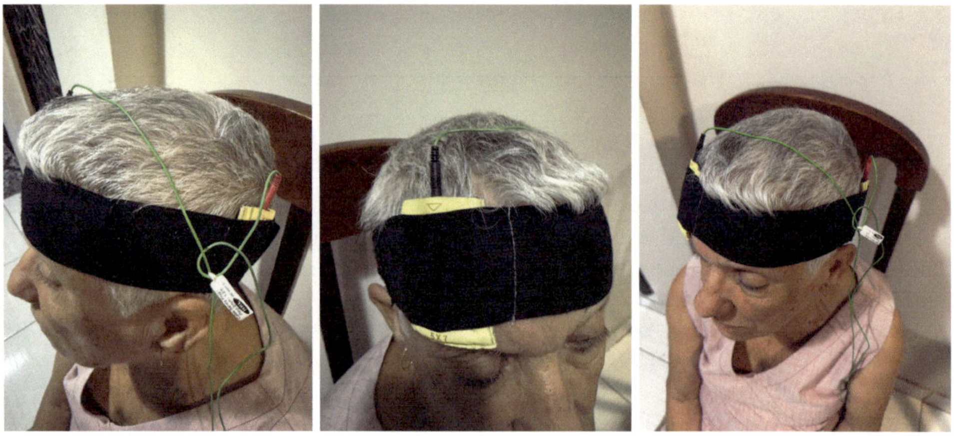

Figure 1.
Photographs of a participant wering a headband with tDCS eletrodes placed on different scalp regions, shown from multiple angles.

contributes to inhibitory processes [15]. tDCS influences the brain's ability to reorganize connections between neurons, a phenomenon known as synaptic plasticity, by modulating neurotransmitters such as glutamate and GABA [24].

Clinical studies and systematic reviews have indicated that tDCS may benefit individuals with depression, stroke, chronic pain, and cognitive deficits, especially when combined with active tasks during stimulation. Reported adverse effects are generally mild and include itching, tingling, or redness at the stimulation site [25].

tDCS has emerged as a promising strategy for managing chronic tinnitus (**Table 2**). Souza et al. (2020) [26] demonstrated that applying tDCS with the anode positioned between T3 and P3 and the cathode at Fp2, according to the EEG 10–20 system, led to a significant reduction in tinnitus perception and

Author/Year [Ref]	Sample/Study type	Protocol	Main findings
Souza et al., 2020 [26]	24 patients; double-blind RCT	Anode T3–P3, cathode Fp2; 2 mA; 5 sessions	Significant reduction in severity and distress; EEG changes observed
Cardon et al., 2022 [29]	77 patients; RCT (HD-tDCS)	Left temporal + right DLPFC; 6 sessions	No significant difference vs. sham; strong placebo effect
Mares et al., 2022 [30]	39 patients	Bifrontal (DLPFC); 6 sessions over 2 weeks	Delayed positive effect lasting up to 6 months
Rashidi et al., 2023 [31]	40 patients; RCT	Bilateral auditory stimulation; 3 weeks	Preliminary results suggest clinical improvement; study ongoing
Repeated Bilateral tDCS, 2024 [32]	48 patients; chronic tinnitus	Bilateral auditory areas; 2 mA; 2 weeks	Significant reduction in THI, VAS, and distress
Lee et al., 2025 [33]	Clinical study	tDCS + counseling; varied protocols	Greater efficacy when combined with counseling, especially in cases of anxiety

Table 2.
Studies on tDCS in tinnitus.

distress. Moreover, it modulated cortical electrical activity in regions involved in sensory-emotional integration and auditory processing compared to placebo.

Lee (2019) [27] investigated tDCS applied to the F3 and F4 regions in patients with tinnitus associated with emotional disturbances. The results indicated that tDCS could modulate cortical circuits related to auditory processing and emotional regulation, including anxiety and depression, particularly in the prefrontal cortex, resulting in approximately a 50% reduction in Tinnitus Handicap Inventory (THI) scores, while the group receiving conventional treatment showed less significant improvement.

Additionally, stimulation of the dorsolateral prefrontal cortex (DLPFC) has shown efficacy in reducing both tinnitus perception and emotional and cognitive symptoms, reinforcing the DLPFC's central role in the affective and attentional regulation of tinnitus [28].

5.1.3 Transcranial random noise stimulation (trns)

Transcranial Random Noise Stimulation (tRNS) involves the application of low-intensity currents through electrodes placed on the scalp (**Figure 2**). It uses an alternating current with randomly varying frequencies, typically ranging from 0.1 Hz to 640 Hz [34, 35].

The central mechanism believed to underlie tRNS is **stochastic resonance**, in which controlled noise facilitates the detection and transmission of weak neural signals, modulating cortical excitability, enhancing neuroplasticity, and promoting the reorganization of brain networks. Although its effects are temporary, they can induce short- or medium-term plastic modifications [34, 36].

There are different variants of the technique:

- **Low-frequency tRNS (lf-tRNS):** Approximately 0.1 to 100 Hz, acts near the physiological rhythms of theta, alpha, and beta waves.

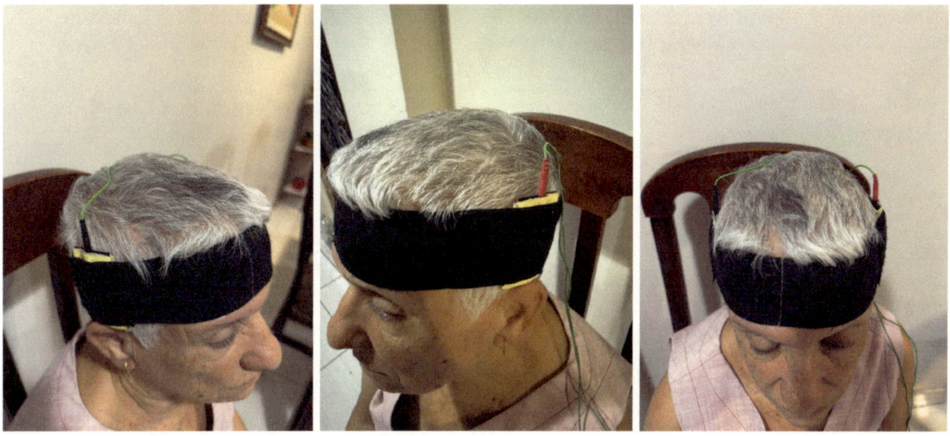

Figure 2.
Photographs of a participant wearing a headband with tRNS electrodes positioned on different scalp regions, shown from multiples angles.

- **High-frequency tRNS (hf-tRNS):** Ranges from 100 to 640 Hz and has been shown to be more effective in increasing cortical excitability and inducing synaptic plasticity by interfering with endogenous oscillations, acting more synchronously on the cortex.

- **Whole-spectrum tRNS:** Covers the entire frequency range from 0.1 to 640 Hz, combining low and high frequencies in a single protocol. It offers broader modulatory effects, though with less consistent outcomes.

In the context of tinnitus, several high-quality clinical studies have reported significant benefits, indicating that tRNS can produce immediate reductions in both loudness and distress associated with the symptom (**Table 3**) [35].

Joos, De Ridder, and Vanneste [37] investigated the effects of transcranial random noise stimulation at different frequency ranges (hf-tRNS and lf-tRNS) in the treatment of tinnitus. The results showed that both modalities reduced symptom intensity, though with distinct effects: hf-tRNS was more effective in patients with pure-tone tinnitus, while lf-tRNS yielded better outcomes in reducing associated distress. These findings reinforce tRNS as one of the most promising noninvasive electrical stimulation techniques, especially in high-frequency and repeated-session protocols.

5.1.4 Transcutaneous auricular vagus nerve stimulation (tavns)

Transcutaneous auricular vagus nerve stimulation (taVNS) is a non-invasive neuromodulation technique that delivers mild electrical impulses to the auricular pavilion in areas with greater vagus nerve innervation, or to the cervical region (**Figure 3**), where the nerve is more superficial and accessible [38].

Stimulation of the vagus nerve activates the nucleus of the solitary tract (NTS), located in the brainstem, which is responsible for integrating visceral and autonomic

Author/Year [Ref]	Sample/Study type	Protocol	Main findings
Vanneste et al., 2013 [42]	111 patients; comparative study	tRNS vs tDCS vs. tACS; one bilateral session	tRNS most effective in immediate reduction of loudness and distress
Claes et al., 2014 [43]	228 patients; retrospective	Single session vs. multiple sessions	Multiple sessions amplified effects, especially on loudness
Joos et al., 2015 [44]	154 patients	lf-tRNS (0.1–100 Hz) vs. hf-tRNS (100–640 Hz)	hf-tRNS reduced loudness in pure tone tinnitus; lf-tRNS reduced distress
Mohsen et al., 2019 [45]	~32 patients; RCT	Multiple cortical targets; multiple sessions	Significant improvement in loudness and annoyance; well-tolerated
Kreuzer et al., 2019 [46]	30 patients; pilot study	hf-tRNS; 2 mA; 10 sessions	Clinical response in 27–31%; no robust effect after correction
Alashram et al., 2024 [47]	Systematic review; 7 studies	616 patients; various protocols	Overall efficacy in reducing loudness/ distress; technique deemed safe

Table 3.
Summary of clinical studies evaluating tRNS for tinnitus, including study design, sample size, stimulation protocols, and main outcomes.

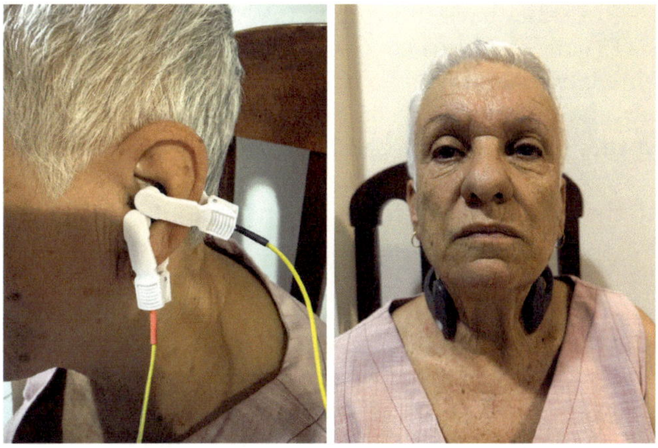

Figure 3.
Photographs of a participant receiving taVNS, showing eletrode placement at the auricular pavilion and cervical region.

signals. In the central nervous system, the NTS connects to structures such as the locus coeruleus, hippocampus, amygdala, thalamus, and prefrontal cortex, promoting synaptic plasticity and modulation of neural networks [39, 40]. Additionally, taVNS influences the autonomic nervous system by increasing parasympathetic activity and regulating physiological parameters such as heart rate variability (HRV) [41].

Controlled clinical trials and systematic reviews have demonstrated the efficacy of taVNS in neurological and psychiatric disorders, such as anxiety disorders, insomnia, and chronic pain (**Table 4**). It is considered a safe and well-tolerated technique, with mild adverse effects such as tingling or itching at the stimulation site [42, 43].

Auricular vagus nerve stimulation (taVNS) facilitates excitation (nucleus of the solitary tract, locus coeruleus, thalamus, cerebellum, insula, and frontal gyrus) or inhibition (amygdala, hippocampus, and parahippocampal gyri) of central circuits involved in tinnitus. Both experimental and clinical studies suggest that taVNS can reduce tinnitus intensity and distress, as well as alleviate comorbid symptoms such as anxiety and stress, thereby expanding therapeutic possibilities for patients with refractory tinnitus [44].

Author/Year [Ref]	Sample/Type	Protocol	Main findings
Kreuzer et al., 2014 (Neuromodulation) [45]	Pilot; few patients	Auricular taVNS (concha)	Feasible and safe technique; trend toward improvement
Yakunina, Kim, and Nam, 2018 (PLoS ONE) [46]	36 patients; fMRI	taVNS at tragus and concha	Activation of locus coeruleus and NTS; deactivation of auditory/limbic areas
Raj-Koziak et al., 2024 (Audiol Neurootol) [47]	29 patients; RCT	taVNS + sound (12 weeks)	No significant clinical improvement; increased theta activity on EEG
Rezapour et al., 2024 (Neurosci. Lett.) [48]	Experimental study in rats	Isolated taVNS	Reduced salicylate-induced tinnitus; improved mood/social behavior

Table 4.
Studies on tavns in tinnitus.

Functional MRI studies have shown that taVNS activates the nucleus of the solitary tract (NTS) and the locus coeruleus, which are critical for norepinephrine release. This stimulation also increases activity in cortical and subcortical regions such as the prefrontal cortex, hippocampus, amygdala, and thalamus – areas associated with auditory perception and the emotional component of tinnitus. Electrode placement in the cymba conchae and tragus regions has shown greater benefits in both the activation and deactivation of tinnitus-related cortical areas.

5.1.5 Photobiomodulation (PBM)

PBM uses low-intensity light in the range of 600 to 810 nm, emitted by LEDs or lasers, with a low power output that avoids thermal effects and is capable of modulating beneficial biochemical responses in neural tissues [49]. One of its main mechanisms of action is on the mitochondrial respiratory chain, specifically the cytochrome c oxidase enzyme. Upon absorbing photons, this enzyme increases ATP production in the mitochondria, reduces oxidative stress, and modulates local inflammation, thereby supporting synaptic plasticity and functional connectivity between brain regions [50]. (**Figure 4**)

PBM can enhance cerebral perfusion, improve tissue oxygenation, and modulate cortical excitability, including in subcortical structures. It alters neural networks relevant to cognitive, emotional, and sensory functions [51].

Recent clinical trials and systematic reviews indicate that PBM has therapeutic potential in conditions such as mild cognitive impairment, depression, chronic pain, and sleep disorders (**Table 5**) [52].

Scheffer et al. (2021) [53] conducted a literature review on scientific output in photobiomodulation, highlighting the growth of publications related to hearing loss and tinnitus.

Masry et al. (2021) [54] evaluated the effectiveness of PBM in patients with bilateral tinnitus and sensorineural hearing loss. The average tinnitus intensity on the visual analog scale (VAS) decreased from 8.0 before treatment to 5.3 after 6 months, suggesting significant clinical improvement.

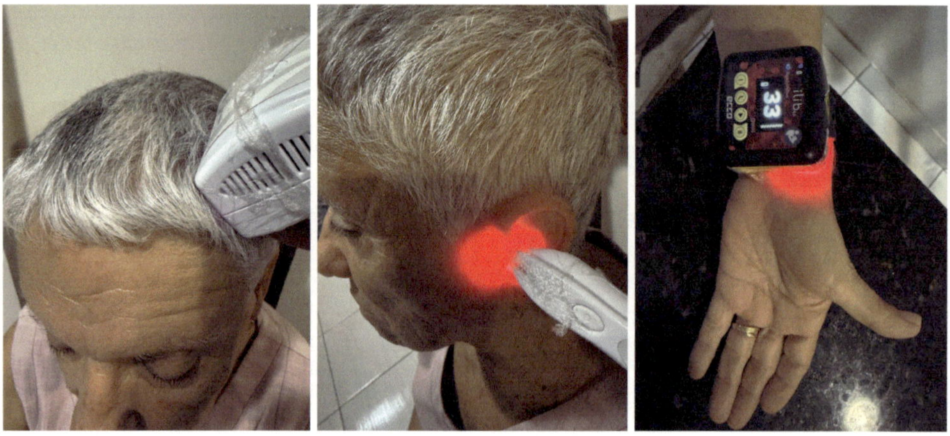

Figure 4.
Photographs of a participant undergoing photobiomodulation, showing transcranial, intracanal, and ILIB applications.

Author/Year [Ref]	Sample/Type	Protocol	Main findings
Cuda and De Caria, 2008 (Int. Tinnitus J.) [53]	Comparative clinical study	PBM + TRT vs. TRT alone	Combined group showed greater reduction in distress and emotional impact
Scheffer et al., 2021 (Int. Tinnitus J.) [54]	Bibliometric review	Scientific output on PBM	Marked increase in studies on hearing loss and tinnitus
Masry et al., 2021 (Int. Arch. Otorhinolaryngol.) [55]	RCT; patients with bilateral tinnitus	Bilateral PBM; 6-month follow-up	VAS decreased from 8.0 → 5.3; significant clinical improvement

Table 5.
Summary clinical and review studies evaluating photobiomodulation (PBM) for tinnitus, incluing study design, treatment protocols, and main outcomes.

Cuda and De Caria (2008) [55] investigated the association between PBM and Tinnitus Retraining Therapy (TRT) in patients with chronic tinnitus, showing that the combination was more effective than TRT alone, with a greater reduction in discomfort and emotional distress.

The concept of multimodal neuromodulation techniques has emerged as a promising alternative to enhance the treatment of chronic tinnitus. The combination of methods (rTMS, tDCS, tRNS, taVNS, PBM) allows for the exploration of complementary mechanisms of neural modulation, thereby increasing the likelihood of a clinical response.

Combining techniques operate at multiple levels of brain plasticity. For example, rTMS and tDCS directly influence cortical excitability and synaptic reorganization in auditory and prefrontal areas by modulating the balance between excitatory and inhibitory neurotransmitters. The integration of these stimuli can generate additive or synergistic effects, facilitating the induction of long-term potentiation or depression in neural networks disrupted by tinnitus.

tRNS, by promoting stochastic resonance, can enhance the detection of weak neural signals, serving as a basal modulator that amplifies the effects of more targeted techniques such as rTMS or tDCS. Vagal stimulation (taVNS) adds an autonomic and limbic component to the process, strengthening connectivity between subcortical and cortical structures involved in tinnitus perception and its emotional impact. PBM contributes through metabolic and anti-inflammatory mechanisms, increasing cellular energy availability and cerebral perfusion, which may facilitate the plastic response induced by other neuromodulation modalities.

Preliminary clinical trials suggest that combining rTMS and tDCS enhances cortical excitability modulation compared to the isolated use of each technique, indicating a synergistic effect on auditory and prefrontal networks. Similarly, the integration of PBM with cognitive therapies or auditory rehabilitation has proven more effective than isolated interventions, highlighting that such combinations support the functional reorganization of both auditory and non-auditory circuits. These findings reinforce the notion that multimodal protocols can more robustly and durably alter neural patterns, thereby increasing therapeutic efficacy and clinical response rates in individuals with chronic tinnitus.

6. Conclusion

Neuromodulation occupies a strategic position in the management of tinnitus, as it targets the neural circuits underlying both perception and distress. By adjusting excitability, synchronization, and synaptic plasticity in auditory and non-auditory networks, these techniques reduce the persistence of the internal signal and attenuate limbic and attentional responses that amplify suffering. Top-down modulation via the DLPFC and ACC, reconfiguration of the DMN, SN, and CEN networks, and neurochemical rebalancing form the core of its therapeutic effects.

Findings from rTMS, tDCS, tRNS, taVNS, and photobiomodulation demonstrate that targeted interventions on cortical and subcortical areas can modify maladaptive neural patterns and promote habituation. Combined protocols tend to enhance clinical outcomes by leveraging complementary mechanisms, uniting excitability modulation, metabolic facilitation, and autonomic and affective regulation. This integrative approach increases the likelihood of clinical response and sustains benefits beyond the stimulation period.

To move forward, it is necessary to standardize parameters, define responder profiles, and integrate neuromodulation with audiological and psychobehavioral strategies. As a therapeutic axis, neuromodulation offers a consistent pathway to reorganize brain networks involved in tinnitus and improve clinical outcomes, particularly in chronic and treatment-resistant cases. However, more high-quality research, especially randomized, double-blind studies, is needed to refine protocols, establish effective combinations, and guide individualized strategies tailored to tinnitus subtypes and the specific needs of each patient.

Author details

Thiago Silva Almeida de Souza[1*] and Lisiane Holdefer[2]

1 Master of Health Sciences, University of São Paulo – USP Brasília, Brasília, Brazil

2 Master and PhD in Medical Sciences, University of Brasília – UnB, Brasília, Brazil

*Address all correspondence to: thiago.fonoaudiologo@gmail.com

References

[1] Jarach CM, Lugo A, Scala M, van den Brandt Pa, Cederroth CR, Odone A, van den Brandt PA, Garavello W, Schlee W, Langguth B, Gallus S. Global prevalence and incidence of tinnitus: A systematic review and meta-analysis. JAMA Neurology. 2022;**79**(9):888–900

[2] Zhang D, Xu Q, Caimino C, Baguley DM. The prevalence of tinnitus in China: A systematic review of the literature. The Journal of Laryngology & Otology. 2021;**135**(1):3–9. DOI: 10.1017/S002221512000256X

[3] De Ridder D, et al. Tinnitus and the Triple Network Model: A perspective. Frontiers in Systems Neuroscience. 2022;**16**:17

[4] Xiong B, Liu Z, Li J, Huang X, Yang J, Xu W, Chen YC, Cai Y, Zheng Y. Abnormal Functional Connectivity Within Default Mode Network and Salience Network Related to Tinnitus Severity. Journal of the Association for Research in Otolaryngology. 2023;**24**(4):453–462. DOI: 10.1007/s10162-023-00905-2

[5] Wang H, Brozoski TJ, Turner JG, Ling L, Parrish JL, Hughes LF, Caspary DM. Plasticity at glycinergic synapses in the dorsal cochlear nucleus of rats with behavioral evidence of tinnitus. Neuroscience. 2009;**164**(2):747–759

[6] Miranda V, Castiglioni S, Maier JA. Neuroplasticity and tinnitus: The role of Brain-Derived Neurotrophic Factor in pathogenesis and treatment. Frontiers in Neuroscience. 2025;**19**:1620894. DOI: 10.3389/fnins.2025.1620894

[7] Sedley W, Friston KJ, Gander PE, Kumar S, Griffiths TD. An integrative tinnitus model based on sensory precision. Trends in Neurosciences. 2016;**39**(12):799–812

[8] Han BI, Lee HW, Kim TY, Lim JS, Shin KS. Tinnitus: Characteristics, causes, mechanisms, and treatments. Journal of Clinical Neurology. 2009;**5**(1):11–19

[9] Shore SE. Mechanisms of noise-induced tinnitus: Insights and clinical implications. Neuroscience and Biobehavioral Reviews. 2019;**96**:13–24

[10] Berboth S, et al. Amygdala-prefrontal connectivity during emotion regulation. Neuroscience Letters. 2021;**760**:136085

[11] Song JJ, De Ridder D, Schlee W, Vanneste S. Dysfunctional noise cancelling of the rostral anterior cingulate cortex in tinnitus patients. Brain. 2015;**138**(3):654–662

[12] Ralli M, Greco A, Altissimi G, Turchetta R, Longo L, de Vincentiis M. Somatosensory tinnitus: Current evidence and future perspectives. Frontiers in Neuroscience. 2017;**11**:207

[13] Wadhwa S, Jain S, Patil N, Jungade S. Cervicogenic Somatic Tinnitus: A Narrative Review Exploring Non-otologic Causes. Cureus. 2024;**16**(7):e65476. DOI: 10.7759/cureus.65476

[14] Lefaucheur JP, Aleman A, Baeken C, et al. Evidence-based guidelines on the therapeutic use of repetitive transcranial magnetic stimulation (rTMS). Clinical Neurophysiology 2020;**131**:474–528

[15] Woods AJ, Antal A, Bikson M, et al. A technical guide to tDCS, and related

non-invasive brain stimulation tools. Clinical Neurophysiology 2016;**127**:1031–1048

[16] Ashton H, Reid K, Marsh R, Johnson I, Alter K, Griffiths T. High frequency localised "hot spots" in temporal lobes of patients with intractable tinnitus: A quantitative electroencephalographic (QEEG) study. Neuroscience Letters. 2007;**426**(1):23–28. DOI: 10.1016/j.neulet.2007.08.034

[17] Khedr EM, Abo-Elfetoh N, Rothwell JC, El-Atar A, Sayed E, Khalifa H. Contralateral versus ipsilateral rTMS of temporoparietal cortex for the treatment of chronic unilateral tinnitus: Comparative study. European Journal of Neurology. 2010;**17**(7):976–983. DOI: 10.1111/j.1468-1331.2010.02965.x

[18] Khedr EM, Rothwell JC, Ahmed MA, El-Atar A. Effect of daily repetitive transcranial magnetic stimulation for treatment of tinnitus: Comparison of different stimulus frequencies. Journal of Neurology, Neurosurgery, and Psychiatry. 2008;**79**(2):212–215. DOI: 10.1136/jnnp.2007.127712

[19] Plewnia C, Vonthein R, Wasserka B, Arfeller C, Naumann A, Schraven SP, Plontke SK. Treatment of chronic tinnitus with θ burst stimulation: A randomized controlled trial. Neurology. 2012;**78**(21):1628–1634. DOI: 10.1212/WNL.0b013e3182574ef9

[20] Folmer RL, Theodoroff SM, Casiana L, Shi Y, Griest S, Vachhani J, et al. Repetitive transcranial magnetic stimulation treatment for chronic tinnitus: A randomized clinical trial. JAMA Otolaryngology–Head & Neck Surgery 2015;**141**:716–722

[21] Landgrebe M, Hajak G, Wolf S, Padberg F, Fallgatter AJ, Rupprecht R, et al. 1-Hz rTMS in the treatment of tinnitus: A sham-controlled, randomized multicenter trial. Brain Stimulation 2017;**10**:1112–1120

[22] Liang Z, Yang H, Cheng G, Huang L, Zhang T, Jia H. Repetitive transcranial magnetic stimulation on chronic tinnitus: A systematic review and meta-analysis. BMC Psychiatry. 2020;**20**(1):547. DOI: 10.1186/s12888-020-02947-9

[23] Nitsche MA, Paulus W. Excitability changes induced in the human motor cortex by weak transcranial direct current stimulation. The Journal of Physiology. 2000;**527**(3):633–639

[24] Fritsch B, Reis J, Martinowich K, et al. Direct current stimulation promotes BDNF-dependent synaptic plasticity: Potential implications for motor learning. Neuron 2010;**66**: 198–204

[25] Dedoncker J, Brunoni AR, Baeken C, Vanderhasselt MA. A systematic review and meta-analysis of the effects of tDCS over the dorsolateral prefrontal cortex in healthy and neuropsychiatric samples. Brain Stimulation. 2016;**9**(4):501–517

[26] Fritsch B, Reis J, Martinowich K, Schambra HM, Ji Y, Cohen LG, Lu B. Direct current stimulation promotes BDNF-dependent synaptic plasticity: Potential implications for motor learning. Neuron. 2010;**66**(2):198–204. DOI: 10.1016/j.neuron.2010.03.035

[27] Lee HY. Adjunctive role of bifrontal tDCS in distressed patients with severe tinnitus. Journal of Korean Medical Science. 2019;**34**(3):e19

[28] Shekhawat GS, Vanneste S. Optimization of tDCS of dorsolateral

prefrontal cortex for tinnitus: A non-linear dose-response effect. Scientific Reports. 2018;**8**(1):8311

[29] Lee HY. Adjunctive Role of Bifrontal Transcranial Direct Current Stimulation in Distressed Patients with Severe Tinnitus. Journal of Korean Medical Science. 2019;**34**(3):e19. DOI: 10.3346/jkms.2019.34.e19

[30] Shekhawat GS, Vanneste S. Optimization of Transcranial Direct Current Stimulation of Dorsolateral Prefrontal Cortex for Tinnitus: A Non-Linear Dose- Response Effect. Scientific Reports. 2018;**8**(1):8311. DOI: 10.1038/s41598-018-26665-1

[31] Souza DDS, Almeida AA, Andrade SMDS, Machado DGDS, Leitão M, Sanchez TG, Rosa MRDD. Transcranial direct current stimulation improves tinnitus perception and modulates cortical electrical activity in patients with tinnitus: A randomized clinical trial. Neurophysiologie Clinique. 2020;**50**(4):289–300. DOI: 10.1016/j.neucli.2020.07.002

[32] Repeated bilateral transcranial direct current stimulation for chronic tinnitus. ClinicalTrials.gov [Internet]. 2024. Available from: https://clinicaltrials.gov [Accessed: 2025-January-10]

[33] Mares T, Albrecht J, Buday J, Podgorna G, Le TH, Magyarova E, Poshor K, Halik J, Buna J, Capek V, Kostylkova L, Klasova J, Fabian V, Anders M. Long-term effect of transcranial direct current stimulation in the treatment of chronic tinnitus: A randomized, placebo-controlled trial. Frontiers in Psychiatry. 2022;**13**:969800. DOI: 10.3389/fpsyt.2022.969800

[34] Terney D, Chaieb L, Moliadze V, Antal A, Paulus W. Increasing human brain excitability by transcranial high-frequency random noise stimulation. The Journal of Neuroscience. 2008;**28**(52):14147–14155

[35] Vanneste S, Fregni F, De Ridder D. Head-to-head comparison of transcranial random noise stimulation, transcranial AC stimulation, and transcranial DC stimulation for tinnitus. Frontiers in Psychiatry. 2013;**4**:158

[36] Fertonani A, Miniussi C. Transcranial electrical stimulation: What we know and do not know about mechanisms. The Neuroscientist. 2017;**23**(2):109–123

[37] Joos K, De Ridder D, Vanneste S. The differential effect of low- versus high-frequency random noise stimulation in the treatment of tinnitus. Experimental Brain Research. 2015;**233**(5):1433–1440

[38] Clancy JA, Mary DA, Witte KK, et al. Non-invasive vagus nerve stimulation in healthy humans reduces sympathetic nerve activity. Brain Stimulation 2014;**7**:871–877

[39] Kaniusas E, Kampusch S, Tittgemeyer M, et al. Current directions in the auricular vagus nerve stimulation I – A physiological perspective. Frontiers in Neuroscience. 2019;**13**:854

[40] Redgrave JN, Day D, Leung H, et al. Safety and tolerability of transcutaneous vagus nerve stimulation in humans: A systematic review. Brain Stimulation 2018;**11**:1225–1233

[41] Joos K, De Ridder D, Vanneste S. The differential effect of low- versus

high-frequency random noise stimulation in the treatment of tinnitus. Experimental Brain Research. 2015;**233** (5):1433–1440. DOI: 10.1007/s00221-015-4217-9

[42] Vanneste S, De Ridder D. Noninvasive and invasive neuromodulation for the treatment of tinnitus: an overview. Neuromodulation. 2012;**15**(4):350-60. DOI: 10.1111/j.1525-1403.2012.00447.x

[43] Claes L, Stamberger H, Van de Heyning P, De Ridder D, Vanneste S. Auditory cortex tACS and tRNS for tinnitus: single versus multiple sessions. Neural Plasticity. 2014;**2014**:436713. DOI: 10.1155/2014/436713

[44] Yakunina N, Nam EC. Direct and transcutaneous vagus nerve stimulation for treatment of tinnitus: A scoping review. Frontiers in Neuroscience. 2021;**15**:680590

[45] Mohsen S, Pourbakht A, Farhadi M, Mahmoudian S. The efficacy and safety of multiple sessions of multisite transcranial random noise stimulation in treating chronic tinnitus. Brazilian Journal of Otorhinolaryngology. 2020;**86**(4):425–433. DOI: 10.1016/j.bjorl.2018.05.010

[46] Yakunina N, Kim SS, Nam EC. Optimization of transcutaneous vagus nerve stimulation using functional MRI. PLoS One. 2018;**13**(3): e0193027

[47] Alashram AR. Computerized cognitive rehabilitation for patients with traumatic brain injury: A systematic review of randomized controlled trials. Applied Neuropsychology: Adult. 2026;**33** (2):578–587. DOI: 10.1080/23279095.2024.2350607

[48] Clancy JA, Mary DA, Witte KK, Greenwood JP, Deuchars SA, Deuchars J. Non-invasive vagus nerve stimulation in healthy humans reduces sympathetic nerve activity. Brain Stimulation. 2014;**7** (6):871–877. DOI: 10.1016/j.brs.2014.07.031

[49] Kaniusas E, Kampusch S, Tittgemeyer M, Panetsos F, Gines RF, Papa M, Kiss A, Podesser B, Cassara AM, Tanghe E, Samoudi AM, Tarnaud T, Joseph W, Marozas V, Lukosevicius A, Ištuk N, Šarolić A, Lechner S, Klonowski W, Varoneckas G, Széles JC. Current Directions in the Auricular Vagus Nerve Stimulation I - A Physiological Perspective. Frontiers in Neuroscience. 2019;**13**:854. DOI: 10.3389/fnins.2019.00854

[50] Redgrave J, Day D, Leung H, Laud PJ, Ali A, Lindert R, Majid A. Safety and tolerability of Transcutaneous Vagus Nerve stimulation in humans; a systematic review. Brain Stimulation. 2018;**11** (6):1225–1238. DOI: 10.1016/j.brs.2018.08.010

[51] Holsboer F, Ros T, Smith RB. Effects of transcranial photobiomodulation on functional connectivity: A randomized, sham-controlled trial. Frontiers in Human Neuroscience. 2025;**19**:1514087

[52] Berman MH, Halper JP, Nichols TW, et al. Photobiomodulation with near infrared light helmet in a pilot, placebo controlled clinical trial in dementia patients. Photomedicine and Laser Surgery 2017;**35**:678–686

[53] Cuda D, De Caria A. Effectiveness of combined counseling and low-level laser stimulation in the treatment of disturbing chronic tinnitus. The

International Tinnitus Journal. 2008;**14**(2):175–180

[54] Scheffer AR, Mfcg M, Rscr T. Photobiomodulation therapy in hearing related aspects: An integrative bibliometric study. The International Tinnitus Journal. 2021;**25**(1):59–65

[55] Masry A, Mahrous AK, El-Samnody AN. Evaluation of low-level laser therapy in bilateral tinnitus with bilateral sensorineural hearing loss. International Archives of Otorhinolaryngology. 2021;**25**(1):e92–e99

Chapter 6

ARC Synaptic Adaptation Therapy: A New Treatment for Tinnitus

Adam Pabiś

Abstract

Tinnitus can be conceptualized as an auditory analogue of phantom pain, where the sudden loss of peripheral input prevents central neural structures from timely reorganization. Clinical evidence indicates that abrupt hearing loss is a major cause of chronic tinnitus, as damage to outer hair cells or auditory nerve fibers leaves the neurons of the spiral ganglion and cochlear nuclei structurally intact but functionally hyperactive. The persistent discharge of these neurons generates the perception of phantom auditory sensations, commonly referred to as tinnitus. By contrast, during gradual hearing loss, neurons undergo *activity-dependent apoptosis* – a natural process of synaptic selection that reduces hyperactivity in response to progressively declining input. Building on this principle, ARC synaptic adaptation therapy is designed to induce activity-dependent apoptosis within the frequency range affected by sudden hearing loss. By applying an acoustic stimulus that gradually decreases in frequency and intensity, the therapy is intended to mimic the conditions of progressive hearing loss, thereby reducing the hyperactive neuronal population and alleviating tinnitus perception. This approach offers a novel therapeutic strategy for targeting the maladaptive neural mechanisms underlying tinnitus.

Keywords: tinnitus, sudden hearing loss, hidden hearing loss, therapy and treatment, neuroplasticity

1. Introduction

Patients with tinnitus commonly describe their condition as a high-pitched tone or a broadband noise perceived within the head. It is estimated tha t approximately 15% of the global population experiences tinnitus, with around 1% of cases associated with significant adverse effects, including depression, anxiety, sleep disturbances, difficulties with concentration, and suicidal thoughts.

According to the 2019 analysis article *Why Is There No Cure for Tinnitus?* (Don J. McFerran [1]), 13 million people worldwide actively seek solutions for the persistent sounds they perceive in their heads. Despite the growing prevalence of tinnitus, including among younger individuals, the field of tinnitus diagnostics and therapy remains limited due to underdeveloped models for clinical recognition and management. To address these challenges, we developed a proprietary method for tinnitus reduction based on extensive clinical experience and scientific knowledge.

The efficacy of this therapy, along with the accompanying diagnostic procedures and patient selection criteria, was subsequently evaluated in a dedicated clinical study.

1.1 Hypothesis and theory – cause and mechanism of tinnitus

It is assumed in this study that the primary cause of tinnitus is the nervous system's inability to adapt to a suddenly occurring hearing loss, resulting in the perception of tinnitus. During gradually progressing hearing loss, the nervous system receives progressively smaller amounts of glutamate released from afferent fibers (**Figure 1**). This gradual reduction in auditory nerve stimulation enables the activation of a neuronal population reduction process, namely apoptosis. The

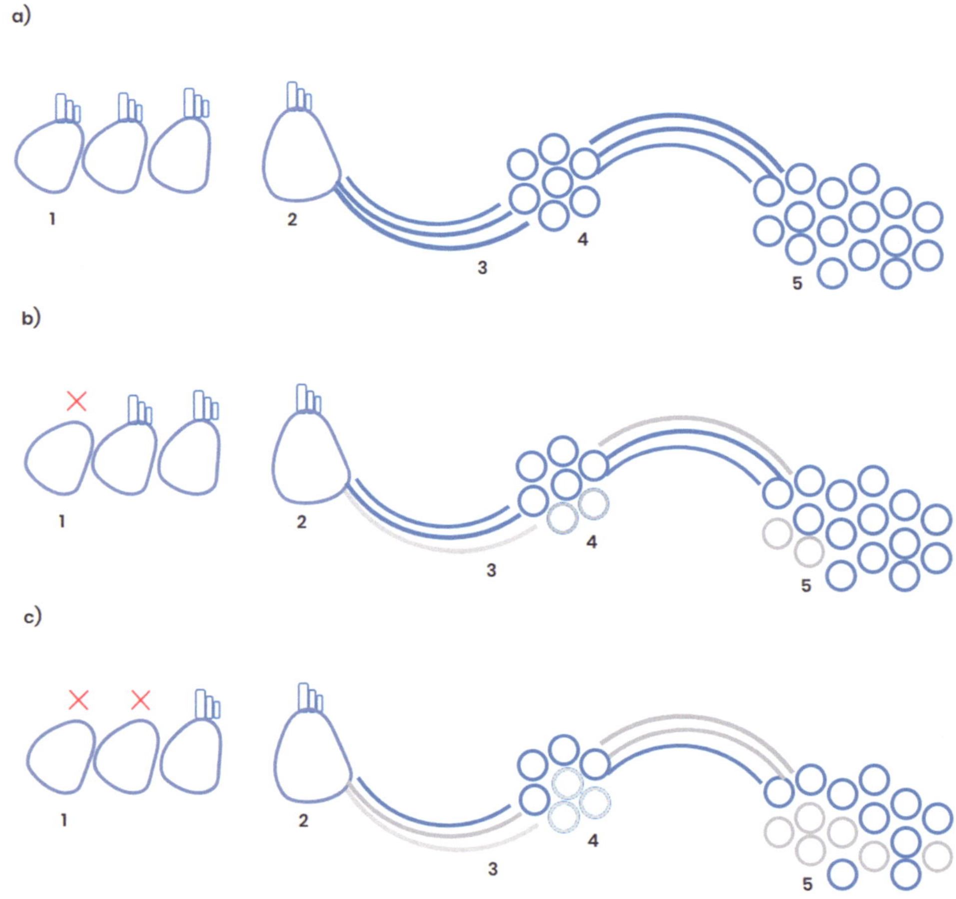

Figure 1.
Schematic representation of the progressive loss of outer hair cells and changes in the number of auditory nerve fibers and neurons.

a) Normal condition – full number of outer hair cells (1) and intact auditory nerve fibers, together with spiral ganglion neurons and cochlear nucleus neurons (3–5).

b) Initial stage of degeneration – loss of individual cells (marked with crosses) and reduction in the number of fibers and neurons (3–5).

c) Advanced stage of degeneration – further loss of outer hair cells and significant removal of some fibers and neurons (3–5).

reduction in neuron numbers serves to adjust the population of nerve cells to the decreased activity of inner hair cells, whose function has been permanently impaired due to damage to outer hair cells within the affected frequency region. By this mechanism, the nervous system does not maintain neurons that fail to process signals, thereby conserving energy.

In cases of sudden hearing loss, the population of neurons in the cochlear nuclei does not undergo significant reduction (**Figure 2**). Outer hair cells die so rapidly that the neurons of the cochlear nuclei cannot initiate apoptosis or natural selection processes, which would otherwise reduce the neuronal population.

Neurons are genetically programmed to regulate their numbers during progressively developing hearing loss. When hearing loss occurs suddenly and the inner hair cells fail to provide stimuli to a neuronal population that has not altered its size or organization, the nervous system may interpret this as a sudden silence in the environment, specifically in the angle of signal incidence and in the spatial region affected by the hearing loss.

Studies have consistently demonstrated an increase in the activity of auditory pathway neurons under conditions of silence (Julien Voisin, Aure´lie Bidet-Caulet [2]).

A statistical increase in constant environmental signals, such as broadband noise, induces a higher rate of neuronal firing, which facilitates more precise and faster analysis of signals, as well as their segregation and spatial grouping. The detection of short-term signals, which may indicate potential threats against the background of slowly varying signals (i.e., background noise), constitutes a crucial component of

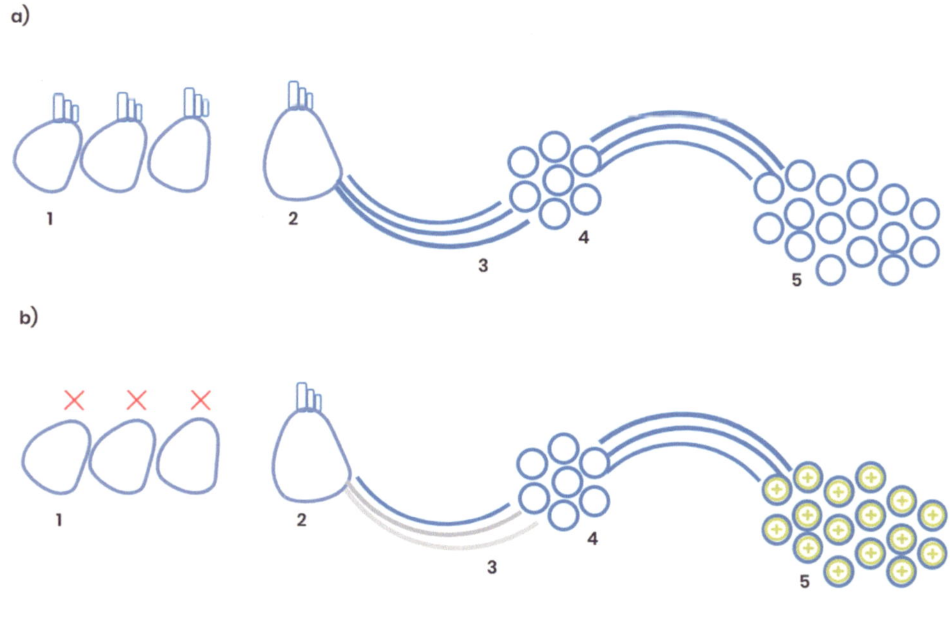

Figure 2.
Schematic representation of the sudden loss of outer hair cells and no change in the number of neurons with increased excitation.

a) Normal condition – full number of outer hair cells (1) and intact auditory nerve fibers with spiral ganglion neurons and cochlear nucleus neurons (3–5).

b) Sudden loss of outer hair cells – and no change in the number of neurons with increased spontaneous excitation (5).

environmental analysis and the perception of safety (Rasmus Kordt Christensen, Florian Studer [3]). In simulated silence induced by sudden hearing loss, the increased firing rate of auditory pathway neurons gives rise to the perception of a sound within the head, which patients describe as tinnitus. Thus, sudden hearing loss effectively simulates an increase in silence within the frequency region where rapid outer hair cell damage has occurred, thereby activating neuronal readiness for faster signal processing.

1.2 The latest research and our theory

Over the past 15 years, hundreds of studies have been conducted with the aim of determining the causes of tinnitus and the correlation between hearing loss and tinnitus. However, most of these studies did not provide a clear answer to the research questions, and a large proportion excluded a relationship between the development of tinnitus and hearing loss. Moreover, practically all of these publications were based on limited pure-tone audiometry up to 8 kHz, which may have limited the ability to detect relationships in higher frequency ranges.

Some studies that examined these frequency ranges reported a direct correlation between hearing loss and tinnitus, particularly in cases of sudden deafness (Ljiljana Cvorovic, Nenad Arsovic [4]). In contrast, the most recent studies (2021–2025), which employed high-frequency pure-tone audiometry from 9 to 20 kHz (for example, see [5–7]) in addition to the standard range (125 Hz–8 kHz), observed a significant difference between patients with tinnitus and the control group. This difference was evident even when the standard frequency range was within normal limits. These findings indicate that damage to cells at very high frequencies is associated with the development of tinnitus and may serve as a clinical marker for its early detection.

Sudden hearing loss does not need to affect a substantial portion of outer hair cells, as is the case in sudden deafness, to activate hyperactivity in auditory pathway neurons.

Indeed, studies have shown that even mild sudden hearing loss, which may not significantly impact auditory perception, can contribute to the generation of tinnitus (Song Z: Tinnitus is associated with extended high-frequency hearing loss [8]).

The scientific literature refers to sudden high-frequency hearing loss as "hidden" because most studies, as well as hearing aid and audiological practices worldwide, assess only up to 8 kHz, rendering hearing deficits in higher frequency ranges – which may contribute to tinnitus – undetectable.

In accordance with our conceptual framework of tinnitus mechanisms, neurons of the cochlear nuclei play a key role in the generation of tinnitus. The increased activity of these neurons, which produces the tinnitus percept, was recorded in the study by James A. Kaltenbach and Donald A. Godfrey [9], thus clearly confirming that heightened excitation of these cells contributes to the generation of the signal perceived by the patient.

Our hypothesis regarding the unchanging structure and number of neurons in the auditory pathway following sudden hearing loss is based on the theory of motor phantom pain observed in patients who have lost limbs. Furthermore, imaging studies from 2025 (Hunter R. Schone, Roni O. Maimon-Mor [10]) demonstrated that, following hand amputation, no significant changes occurred in the structure, organization, or number of neurons, thereby supporting our assumptions concerning the stability of cochlear nucleus neurons after sudden hearing loss.

1.3 Current therapies and their limitations

Specialists worldwide propose a variety of therapeutic strategies for tinnitus, the primary aim of which is to divert attention from the intrusive sound in the head or to effectively mask it. One of the earliest approaches is Cognitive Behavioral Therapy (CBT), which primarily seeks to teach patients not to focus on their tinnitus by modifying emotional and cognitive responses. This method is often combined with the recommendation to listen more frequently to environmental sounds or artificially generated signals.

Another therapeutic approach is tinnitus retraining therapy (TRT), typically applied during the evening and sleep periods when tinnitus is most pronounced. The administered broadband noise is intended to habituate the nervous system to a repetitive stimulus, thereby reducing its subjective perceptibility.

According to the systematic review *Effects of Tinnitus Retraining Therapy on Patients with Tinnitus: A Systematic Review of Randomized Controlled Trials* (Anas R. Alashram [11]), the effectiveness of TRT was comparable to other tinnitus management methods, including masking, education, and CBT.

However, all of these approaches share a significant limitation arising from the lack of updates to fundamental assumptions, procedures, and stimulation protocols in light of contemporary knowledge in neurobiology and neurochemistry. Tinnitus generators still produce signals only up to 8 kHz, excluding patients whose sudden hearing loss and tinnitus locus occur within the 9–20 kHz range.

Hearing aids constitute another available technology demonstrating potential for tinnitus reduction, particularly in patients with hearing loss in the speech comprehension range (125 Hz–12 kHz). The main limitation of this technology is the restricted signal amplification bandwidth, most commonly limited to 7.5–8 kHz. In cases where sudden hearing loss and tinnitus occur within the 4–12 kHz range, the hearing aid does not cover the full necessary bandwidth, thereby limiting the potential for significant symptom reduction.

In recent years, solutions utilizing neuromodulation of neuronal behavior through alternating stimulus delivery – such as sound or somatosensory potentials – have also been developed. This approach demonstrates substantial efficacy only in patients whose tinnitus includes a somatosensory component, reflecting a specific type of neuronal plasticity. Patients exhibiting other plasticity models do not show significant improvement in tinnitus reduction.

1.4 ARC synaptic adaptation therapy – concept and objectives

The nervous system possesses an active strategy that regulates the number of neurons proportionally to the level of signal and stimulation generated by inner hair cells. However, this strategy fails in situations where hair cells undergo sudden damage, resulting in the same population of neurons after the loss as before. A side effect of the lack of a conducted process of neuron number selection for reduction is tinnitus, as perceived by the patient.

Synaptic Adaptation Therapy (ARC) aims to induce a simulated activity-dependent apoptotic process within the frequency range of the inner ear, utilizing a specialized acoustic stimulus algorithm. Administering gradually decreasing acoustic stimulation in both time and intensity to hair cells in the region of sudden damage is intended to replicate processes occurring during.

Gradual hearing loss, including the selection and elimination of unnecessary neurons, ultimately leads to a reduction in tinnitus.

The acoustic stimulus is delivered via a specialized external signal generator connected to in-ear high-frequency headphones, which are open and do not occlude the external auditory canal. The device's controlling software automatically adjusts the intensity and frequency of the signal weekly, gradually reducing both according to settings programmed by a specialist. The frequency range over which the tone algorithm is applied is adjustable from 125 Hz to 20 kHz, allowing stimulation to cover any combination of hearing loss width and depth.

The loudness of each individual tonal signal is independently adjustable across channels, enabling the combination of multiple tones at varying levels, covering different cellular response thresholds across multiple frequencies. The signal perceived by the patient is quiet and barely noticeable, allowing for prolonged use of the stimulation. The device is recommended for 8 hours of daily use, with breaks covering the remaining 16 hours of the day. To achieve therapeutic effects, the stimulation should be administered daily, maintaining the prescribed time regimen.

The application of an artificial environment for controlled sound-induced apoptosis in patients with tinnitus, aimed at regulating the number of midbrain neurons following sudden hearing loss, represents the first such initiative worldwide. Previously, the effect of gradually decreasing acoustic stimulation on tinnitus reduction had not been investigated.

2. Hearing tests performed and patient qualification process for clinical trials

The study included women and men aged 18 to 60 years, all of whom were right-handed. Inclusion criteria required chronic, persistent, non-pulsatile tinnitus lasting no longer than two years, with the exception of two participants who had experienced the symptom for a longer period. Tinnitus could be unilateral or bilateral, and its character could be broadband or tonal.

All participants underwent measurements of serum or plasma levels of serotonin and brain-derived neurotrophic factor (BDNF). Eligible participants had elevated serotonin levels (>100 µg/L) and BDNF levels ranging from 18 to 31 ng/mL. The ratio of HDL to LDL cholesterol was also considered, with a requirement for it to be approximately 1:1 or very close.

Hearing loss affected the 10–20 kHz range and occurred within a model of spontaneous activity plasticity, without observable changes in the reorganization of the tonotopic map of neurons.

Before and during the study, participants were instructed to follow dietary and physical activity recommendations to maintain optimal BDNF levels. Each participant also underwent otoscopy to exclude ear canal obstruction or middle ear infection. Average hearing loss on the audiogram could not exceed 70 dB at any single frequency, and the hearing loss had to appear suddenly within the 10–20 kHz range. Additionally, participants exposed to occupational noise or suffering from depression, anxiety, or sleep disturbances were excluded to ensure a stable study environment and minimize factors that could modulate tinnitus perception.

Previous research indicates that patients with tinnitus tend to have higher blood glucose levels and increased sensitivity to fluctuations (Wenqing Xia, Jinluan Cui [12]). Excess glucose may negatively affect the function of cochlear cells and auditory nerve fibers, contributing to worsening hearing loss and tinnitus severity. Similarly, the HDL-to-LDL ratio plays a role in hearing protection and proper auditory pathway function (Jichang Wu [13]). Considering these factors helps minimize variability in therapeutic outcomes.

The study visit included an audiological interview, questionnaire completion, and a series of audiological assessments. High-frequency pure-tone audiometry was conducted across 125 Hz–20 kHz, along with impedance audiometry and tinnitus-specific tests, including identification of frequencies that suppress tinnitus, otoacoustic emission measurements, and auditory brainstem response (ABR) testing.

Following pure-tone audiometry, a test was conducted to identify frequencies affecting tinnitus perception. Participants were presented with a continuous tone via headphones at their hearing threshold, as determined in audiometry, covering frequencies from low to high (125 Hz–20 kHz). They were asked to indicate whether the tone suppressed their tinnitus or whether it remained audible along with the tone. Testing began with frequency ranges unaffected by hearing loss (125 Hz–10 kHz) and then covered frequencies affected by sudden hearing loss.

Audiogram analysis revealed two characteristic patterns associated with sudden hearing loss. The first was a flat line across several frequencies, corresponding to pantonal hearing loss (**Figure 3**), while the second formed a V– or U-shaped pattern (**Figure 4**).

In the 10–20 kHz range, corresponding to areas of sudden hearing loss, continuous tone presentation was most effective in reducing tinnitus. Patients frequently reported that their tonal tinnitus resembled the sound presented through headphones in the region of hearing loss.

The study was further extended with ipsilateral and contralateral stimulation tests applied to patients with both unilateral and bilateral tinnitus. The objective was to determine whether bilateral tinnitus resulted from sudden hearing loss in both ears or from unilateral hearing loss, in which tinnitus arises due to hyperactivity of the calyx of Held synaptic terminal, generating high-frequency signals on the side opposite the affected ear. In such cases, presenting the signal to one ear suppressed tinnitus in both ears.

2.1 Study group (participants)

A total of 37 individuals diagnosed with tinnitus were enrolled in the study. Of these, 27 participants (72.9%) were assigned to the experimental group receiving acoustic stimulation, while 10 (27.0%) were allocated to the placebo group. Women predominated in the entire sample: 19 women and 8 men were included in the experimental group, whereas the placebo group consisted of 3 women and 7 men. The mean age of the participants was 29.7 ± 5.6 years in the experimental group and 34.5 ± 9.0 years in the placebo group. Overall, the placebo group tended to be slightly older and more male-dominated than the experimental group.

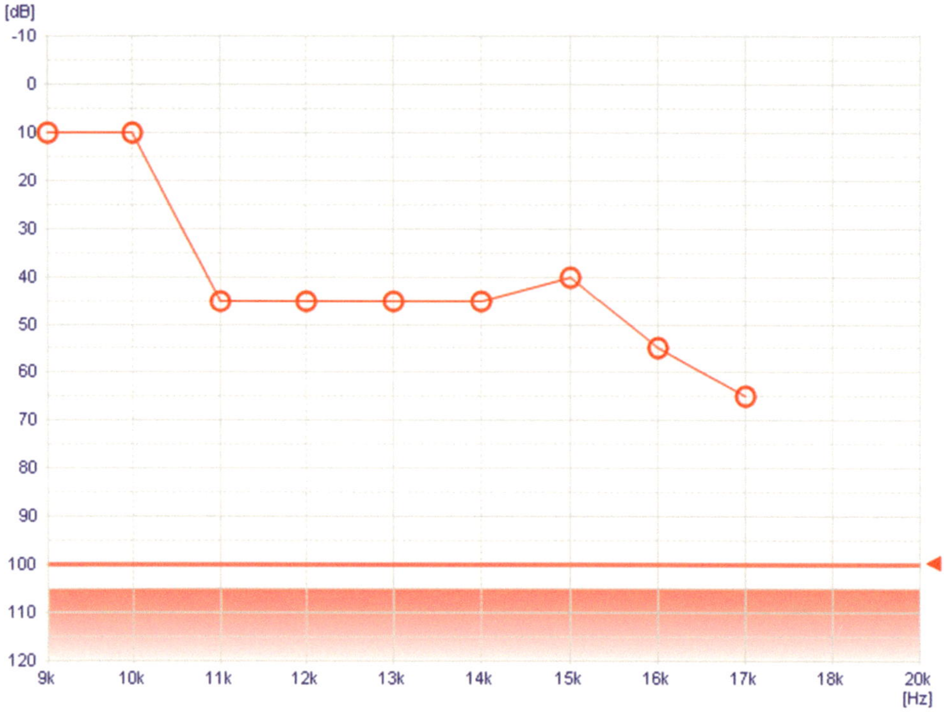

Figure 3.
A high-frequency audiogram and the result in the form of a pantonal flat sudden hearing loss curve in the frequency range from 11 to 15 kHz.

The duration of tinnitus varied among participants. In the experimental group, 40.7% reported the symptom for less than six months, 55.6% for one to two years, and only a few individuals for longer durations.

In contrast, the distribution in the placebo group was different: 10% of participants reported tinnitus lasting less than 6 months, 70% between 1 and 2 years, 10% between 2 and 5 years, and another 10% longer than 5 years. This suggests that, on average, tinnitus duration was somewhat longer in the placebo group.

The mean hearing loss, assessed at high frequencies (8–20 kHz), was 45 dB HL in the experimental group and 37 dB HL in the placebo group. The character of tinnitus also differed: the majority of participants in the experimental group (81.5%) described it as tonal, with 18.5% reporting broadband tinnitus, whereas in the placebo group, these values were 70% and 30%, respectively. Furthermore, perception of tinnitus in the "center of the head" was reported by 92.6% of the experimental group but only 50% of the placebo group, indicating a more homogeneous perception pattern among those receiving the intervention. Tinnitus was more rarely perceived in the right or left ear, and all participants were right-handed.

Selected biological parameters were also assessed. Serum BDNF concentrations ranged from 18.3 to 31.4 ng/mL, while serotonin levels ranged from 80 to 280 ng/mL (minimum and maximum values for the entire sample are reported). Average lipid concentrations in the cohort were 85 mg/dL for HDL and 100 mg/dL for LDL.

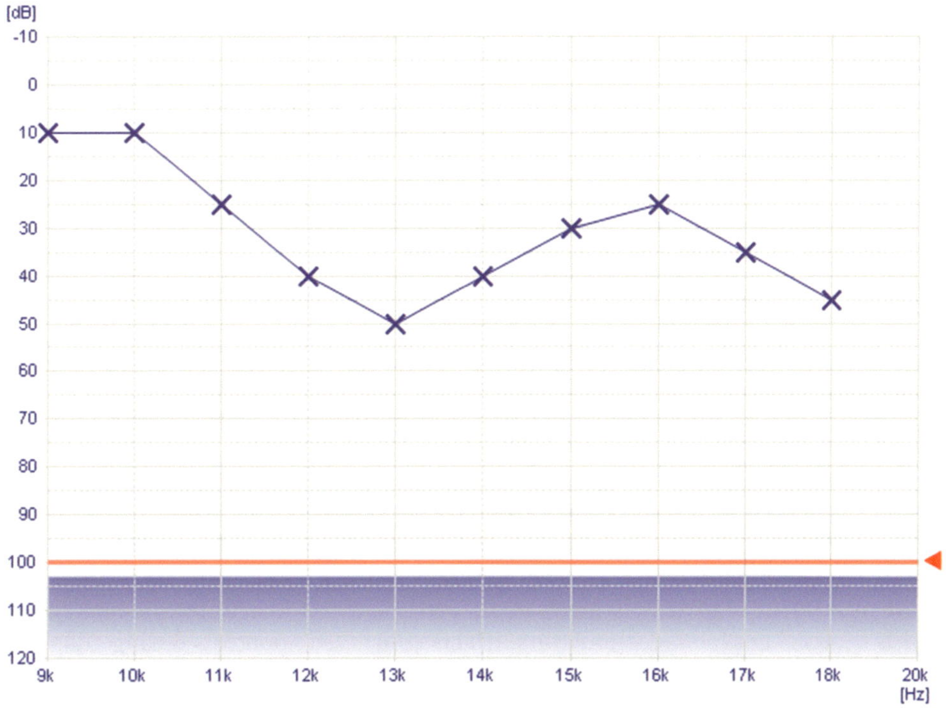

Figure 4.
A high-frequency audiogram and the result in the form of a curve of sudden hearing loss in the shape of a V or U in the frequency range from 11 to 16 kHz.

No relevant between-group differences were observed in these laboratory parameters. The average device usage time was 6.67 ± 1.36 hours per day in the experimental group and 6.3 ± 1.34 hours per day in the placebo group. Throughout the observation period, no serious adverse events related to acoustic stimulation were recorded. Taken together, both groups were broadly comparable in terms of device use and safety, allowing subsequent analyses to be interpreted without confounding effects from adherence or tolerability.

2.2 Brain-derived neurotrophic factor (BDNF) as a marker of treatment effectiveness and a factor qualifying for treatment

Brain-derived neurotrophic factor (BDNF) is a key regulator of the development, survival, and plasticity of neurons within the auditory pathway. In adulthood, across the frequency range from low tones up to 8 kHz, BDNF plays a protective and regenerative role for cochlear cells and auditory nerve fibers following noise-induced or ototoxic damage. Adequate BDNF levels determine how auditory stimuli influence neuronal behavior and the encoding of memory during stimulation and learning.

At the level of the central auditory system, reduced BDNF levels promote the opening of a greater number of calcium channels in presynaptic trapezoid body cells and Calyx of Held synaptic terminals, making them more prone to spontaneous activity. This, in turn, increases neuronal excitability and may contribute to the enhancement of tinnitus perception (Xiaowen Zhuang, Wei Sun, Sascha Lessle, Lena Ebbers, Baydyuk [14–16]). In the cochlear nuclei, appropriate BDNF levels help maintain the balance between excitatory (glutamatergic) and inhibitory (GABAergic) transmission, which is essential for neuronal sensitivity and accurate frequency mapping.

Low BDNF levels also limit neuronal plasticity, which may reduce the effectiveness of external stimuli in modulating neuronal behavior or structure. Consequently, BDNF can serve as a valuable marker of brain plasticity and, by extension, of the potential effectiveness of therapeutic interventions. In our study, BDNF levels were used as a qualification criterion.

Patients with insufficient levels were not eligible to begin the procedure unless they implemented dietary and physical activity recommendations aimed at stimulating BDNF production. Participants with BDNF levels within the range of 18–31 ng/mL were admitted to the procedure. Adequate BDNF levels indicate high neuronal plasticity, increasing the likelihood that auditory stimulation will effectively modulate neuronal function.

Beyond BDNF, future research may consider additional markers to assess the efficacy of tinnitus therapies.

Measurement of proBDNF levels could provide direct insight into the extent to which decreasing acoustic stimulation affects controlled apoptosis during adaptive synaptic therapy (ARC), allowing for the prediction of therapeutic outcomes prior to intervention. We also hypothesize that increasing BDNF levels may reduce hyperactivity within the central auditory pathway, potentially enhancing the effects of both acoustic and neuromodulatory therapies.

2.3 Procedure and selection of acoustic signal – ARC synaptic adaptation therapy

Each participant received an individually programmed signal generator, adjusted to the specific frequencies corresponding to the range associated with sudden hearing loss (10–20 kHz), allowing for precise acoustic stimulation. Both groups underwent stimulation for a period of four months, with the initially rapidly repeating signal being identical in both groups.

In the experimental group, after one week of device use, the software automatically initiated a signal with gradually decreasing repetition frequency over time (5 signals per second in the first week, 3 signals per second in the following week) (**Figure 5**), with the interval between consecutive signals gradually increasing, whereas the placebo group received a constant signal with an unchanging repetition frequency throughout the entire four-month period.

Additionally, in the experimental group, the stimulus intensity was gradually reduced each month, which enhanced the effect of diminishing stimulation and allowed for observation of the impact of the device's adaptive mechanism on sound perception. Two months after the start of stimulation, participants attended a follow-up visit to assess the technical condition of the headphones and connect the device to download data on the frequency and regularity of stimulation use. At the end of the four-month period, participants returned to return the device and completed a questionnaire evaluating the course of therapy and the subjective perception of the stimulation effects.

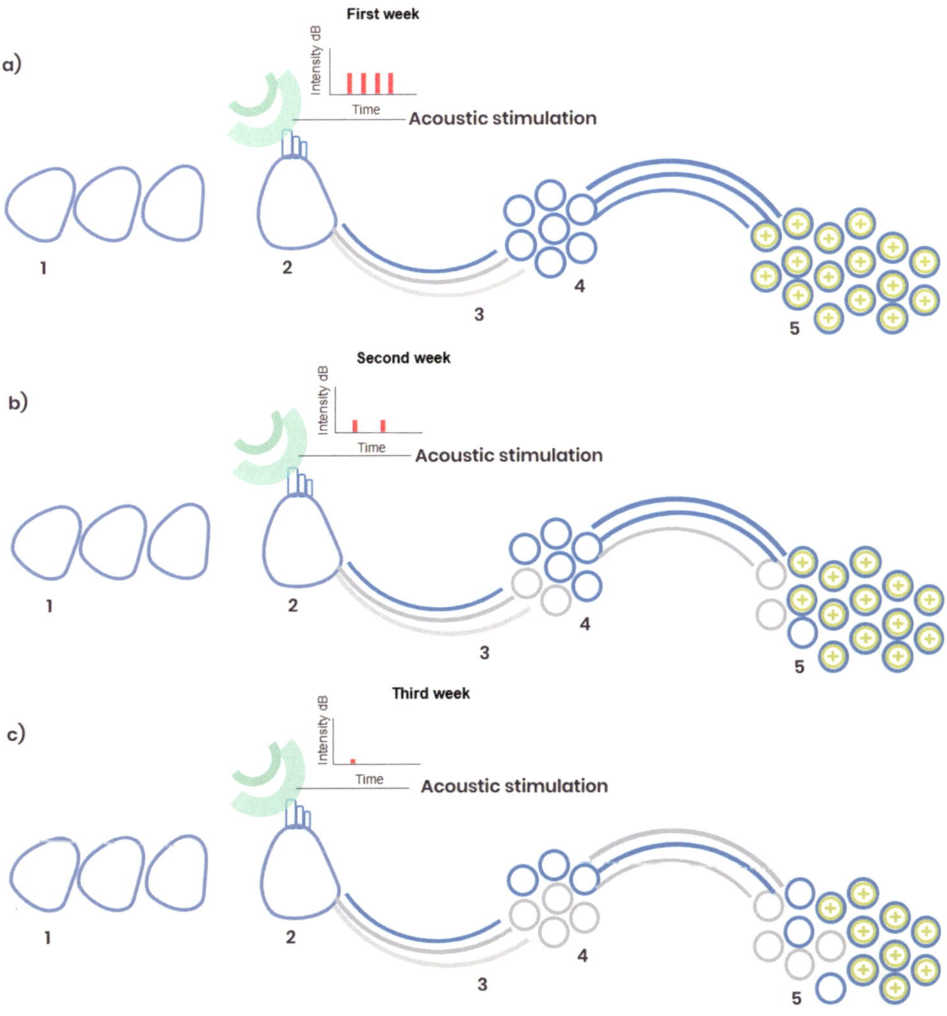

Figure 5.
Progressive reduction of neuronal activity in response to ARC-decreasing acoustic stimulation of the inner hair cell (2).

a) During the first week, repetitive and higher-intensity acoustic stimulation is delivered (inset graph), leading to robust activation of auditory nerve fibers (3), spiral ganglion neurons (4), and a large population of cochlear nucleus neurons (5).

b) In the second week, acoustic stimulation occurs less frequently and with lower intensity, resulting in the activation of the selection process of parts of the auditory nerve (3) fibers and cochlear nucleus neurons (5).

c) By the third week, stimulation is rare and weak, leading to a marked decline in neural activity and a significant reduction in the population of cochlear nucleus neurons (5).

This scheme illustrates the progressive impact of reduced sensory input on neuronal survival and connectivity within the auditory pathway.

2.4 Results

The study results indicate that adaptive synaptic therapy (ARC) produces both statistically significant and clinically meaningful improvements in patients with chronic tinnitus. After four months of therapy, participants in the experimental group (n = 27) reported an average symptom reduction of 64.8%, whereas no improvement was observed in the placebo group (n = 10). Remarkably, 59% of patients in the active group achieved a reduction in tinnitus severity exceeding 70%, confirming the high efficacy of the intervention.

A parallel decrease in subjective tinnitus distress – from 7.85 to 2.15 points on a 0–10 scale – reflects not only improved symptom perception but also a substantial enhancement of participants' comfort and quality of life.

Building on these outcomes, we observed that tinnitus in the experimental group was predominantly perceived as centrally localized, as reported by 92.6% of participants (25 of 27). This type of perceptual topography may reflect the engagement of central auditory processing structures – such as the auditory cortex, thalamus, and integrative networks – in symptom generation. While the therapy was effective in patients with unilateral tinnitus as well, the high proportion of central perception among those showing marked improvement suggests the existence of a subgroup particularly responsive to the neuromodulatory effects of adaptive stimulation.

Thus, central perceptual localization may serve as a practical predictive marker of clinical response and guide further efforts in treatment personalization.

In parallel, the study incorporated measurements of BDNF and serotonin – biomolecules critical for neuroplasticity and auditory processing. The inclusion of these biomarkers provides a link between perceptual outcomes and underlying biological mechanisms, allowing for the identification of correlates of therapeutic efficacy and the development of predictive models for treatment response. Future research should focus on validating these markers in larger populations and determining their utility in forecasting therapeutic outcomes.

The therapy was also found to be completely safe and well-tolerated, with no reported adverse effects. The observed therapeutic effect, occurring across a population diverse in age and sex, underscores the potential for broad application of ARC in routine clinical practice, particularly in the outpatient management of patients with idiopathic, chronic tinnitus.

Contextualizing these findings within current clinical guidelines – such as AAO-HNSF (2014), NICE (2020), and VA/DoD (2024) – reveals a lack of strong, definitive recommendations for causal treatment of tinnitus. Existing guidelines primarily emphasize patient education, symptom management, and psychosocial support. Sound-based, pharmacological, and neuromodulatory therapies remain cautiously recommended, often with conditional or weak endorsements due to the limited number of high-quality clinical studies linking efficacy to mechanisms of action.

In this context, the present study not only provides robust clinical data but also elucidates specific mechanisms underlying ARC stimulation, both in perceptual terms (central tinnitus localization) and biological terms (BDNF, serotonin).

These insights may form the foundation for incorporating personalized acoustic neuromodulation into future clinical recommendations as a targeted therapy based on the patient's neurophysiological profile. Despite the limited sample size and follow-up duration, the results offer a solid basis for further research and clinical validation.

Adaptive synaptic therapy (ARC) represents an innovative, safe, and effective therapeutic approach with high translational potential, integrating clinical personalization with biologically grounded mechanisms of action. Its continued

DOI: http://dx.doi.org/10.5772/intechopen.1013558

validation may not only address an existing therapeutic gap but also contribute to shaping future standards in tinnitus management.

3. The future of ARC synaptic adaptation therapy

ARC synaptic adaptation therapy begins with a precise and extended hearing assessment – tonal audiometry up to 20 kHz. While such measurements are rarely performed in hearing centers and audiology clinics worldwide due to limited specialized equipment, they are essential for tailoring therapy to each patient. Globally, hundreds of millions of people suffer from tinnitus, yet access to effective, individualized therapy remains extremely limited. This scarcity has long restricted access to ARC therapy, creating a real barrier to its wider adoption and global impact. However, by digitizing our solutions alongside the diagnostic procedure, we aim to overcome these limitations and bring this therapy to more people around the world.

3.1 Mobile application

Today, ARC therapy is available only on-site at authorized hearing care centers in Poland. But the vision for the future is global: a solution that reaches patients wherever they are, without the need to travel to a clinic. We are developing a mobile application that guides patients through an automated interview and diagnostic assessment. From there, it designs a fully personalized acoustic stimulation program with the ARC therapy protocol – eliminating the need for an in-person visit.

Creating such an application is no small feat. Translating the precision of high-frequency clinical hearing tests into a mobile format, while integrating automated algorithm selection, requires rigorous validation and testing. Yet, the potential impact is enormous: more patients worldwide can gain access to our expertise, and tinnitus – once a persistent global challenge – could finally become manageable. This represents not just a technological advancement, but a meaningful leap in improving the quality of life for those affected across the globe.

3.2 Hearing aids

Most modern hearing aids amplify specific frequency ranges, but they also often include a built-in tinnitus noise generator. In this mode, patients hear a carefully calibrated sound rather than amplification, with the level and bandwidth adjusted by a hearing care professional.

Looking ahead, we plan to collaborate with hearing aid manufacturers to integrate ARC therapy directly into their devices, much like existing tinnitus noise generators. Historically, this was impossible because most hearing aids limited signal transmission to 7–8 kHz.

Today, however, more devices support broader amplification bandwidths above 8 kHz, opening the door to using hearing aids as full-fledged ARC signal generators. This technological shift has the potential to bring ARC therapy to millions of patients worldwide, making it not only innovative but globally scalable.

By combining cutting-edge diagnostics, mobile technology, and hearing aid integration, ARC therapy is moving from specialized clinics to everyday life around the world. What was once a daunting global problem – tinnitus – may soon become a condition that patients can truly manage, guided by both technology and science.

4. Conclusion

Tinnitus is an exceptionally complex condition that spans multiple disciplines, including audiology, neurobiology, and neurochemistry. Patients enrolled in our study experienced significant therapeutic effects. However, these were individuals who had previously struggled with metabolic imbalances, elevated glucose levels, and low levels of brain-derived neurotrophic factor (BDNF). Following the implementation of an appropriate diet and physical activity protocol, these factors were regulated, creating a stable environment for the introduction of ARC therapy.

The inner ear, auditory nerve, and neurons of the auditory pathway are not isolated structures. The functioning of each tissue depends on factors such as glucose levels, cholesterol, hormones, and minerals. When designing the study, we aimed to prepare patients in a way that would allow for changes in neuronal behavior or structure while minimizing the influence of other negative factors on neural plasticity. Optimizing patients' health and applying appropriate eligibility criteria may be key to the effectiveness of various therapeutic interventions, both current and future.

Multifaceted, gradually decreasing acoustic stimulation used in ARC therapy produced measurable effects in patients with tinnitus. Patients reported that the tinnitus, which had previously been constantly present, became less intrusive, and its perceived loudness significantly decreased. In the experimental group, the average reduction in tinnitus severity was approximately 65% (from 7.85 to 2.15 on a 0–10 scale), whereas no clinically significant improvement was observed in the placebo group.

The therapy was well-tolerated, with no adverse events attributed to the device. These findings suggest that acoustic stimulation, employing a signal that activates processes occurring during gradual hearing loss at the site of sudden onset, may constitute an effective, safe, and non-invasive method to support tinnitus treatment. Patients who had experienced sudden high-frequency hearing loss, in particular, reported improved quality of daily life, as tinnitus no longer dominated their perception of environmental sounds.

Additionally, the study monitored levels of brain-derived neurotrophic factor (BDNF). Increasing evidence indicates that both total BDNF levels and the proBDNF/mBDNF ratio may reflect central nervous system plasticity and correlate with treatment response. Monitoring these parameters in future studies could facilitate personalized treatment, identify patients most likely to respond to acoustic stimulation, and assess the efficacy and durability of therapeutic effects.

Further, larger, and longer-term studies are necessary to confirm these results and to investigate the relationship between clinical improvement and biomarkers such as BDNF and serotonin. At the same time, these findings indicate that ARC Synaptic Adaptation Therapy has the potential to become an innovative tool for tinnitus management, offering patients tangible improvements in quality of life and new therapeutic perspectives.

Author details

Adam Pabiś
Kinetic Center of Advanced Audiology, Warsaw, Poland

*Address all correspondence to: adampabis@kinetic-cna.pl

References

[1] McFerran DJ. Why is there no cure for Tinnitus? Frontiers in Neuroscience. 2019;**13**:2019. DOI: 10.3389/fnins.2019.00802

[2] Voisin J. Aure´lie Bidet-Caulet listening in silence activates auditory areas: A functional magnetic resonance imaging study. The Journal of Neuroscience. 2006;**26**(1):273–278. DOI: 10.1523/JNEUROSCI.2967-05.2006

[3] Christensen RK, Studer F. Background white noise increases neuronal activity by reducing membrane fluctuations and slow-wave oscillations in auditory cortex. Progress in Neurobiology. 2025;**246**:102720. DOI: 10.1016/j.pneurobio.2025.102720

[4] Cvorovic L, Arsovic N. Acute onset of tinnitus in patients with sudden deafness. Noise & Health. 2021;**23** (110):81–86. DOI: 10.4103/nah.NAH_42_20

[5] Vielsmeier V. The relevance of the high frequency audiometry in tinnitus patients with normal pure-tone audiometry. BioMed Research International. 2015:302515. DOI: 10.1155/2015/302515

[6] Ding Z. Extended high-frequency audiometric analyses of tinnitus patients exhibiting normal hearing on conventional PTA (2022). Acta Otolaryngologica. 2022;**142**(7–8): 579–584. DOI: 10.1080/00016489.2022.2112972

[7] Abu-Eta R. Extended high-frequency audiometry for revealing sudden sensorineural hearing loss in acute tinnitus patients. International Archives of Otorhinolaryngology. 2021;**25**(3):e413–e415. DOI: 10.1055/s-0040-1713921

[8] Song Z. Tinnitus is associated with extended high-frequency hearing loss otol neurotol. Otology & Neurotology. 2021;**42**(3):377–383. DOI: 10.1097/MAO.0000000000002983

[9] Kaltenbach JA, Godfrey DA. Dorsal Cochlear Nucleus Hyperactivity and Tinnitus: Are They Related? Journal of the American Academy of Audiology. 2008;**19**(4):293–304. DOI: 10.1044/1059-0889(2008/08-0004)

[10] Schone HR, Maimon-Mor RO, Kollamkulam M, Szymanska MA, Gerrand C, Woollard A, Kang NV, Baker CI, Makin TR. Stable cortical body maps before and after arm amputation. Nature Neuroscience. 2025;**28**:2015–2021. DOI: 10.1038/s41593-025-02037-7

[11] Alashram AR. Effects of Tinnitus retraining therapy on patients with tinnitus: A systematic review of randomized controlled trials. European Archives of Oto-Rhino-Laryngology. 2025;**282**(2):571–87. DOI: 10.1007/s00405-024-08907-3

[12] Xia W, Cui J, Luo Y, Xu -J-J, Chen H, Yin X, Ma J, Wu Y. Glucose control has an impact on cerebral blood flow alterations in chronic tinnitus patients. Frontiers in Neuroscience. 2020;**14**. DOI: 10.3389/fnins.2020.623520

[13] Wu J. Impact of cholesterol homeostasis within cochlear cells on auditory development and hearing loss. Frontiers in Cellular Neuroscience.

2024;**17**:2023. DOI: 10.3389/fncel.2023.1308028

[14] Zhuang X, Sun W, Xu-Friedman MA. Changes in properties of auditory nerve synapses following conductive hearing loss. Journal of Neuroscience. 2017;**37**(2):323–332. DOI: 10.1523/JNEUROSCI.0523-16.2016

[15] Lessle S, Ebbers L. Maintenance of a central high frequency synapse in the absence of synaptic activity. Frontiers in Cellular Neuroscience. 2024;**18**. DOI: 10.3389/fncel.2024.1404206

[16] Baydyuk, et al. Brain-derived neurotrophic factor inhibits calcium channel activation, exocytosis and endocytosis at a central nerve terminal. The Journal of Neuroscience. 2015;**35**(11):4676–4682. DOI: 10.1523/JNEUROSCI.2695-14.2015

Chapter 7

Perspective Chapter: Auditory Rehabilitation in Challenging Cases – Strategies and Outcomes

Cilmara Cristina Alves da Costa Levy

Abstract

The generalization of auditory rehabilitation is not acceptable today, especially considering the significant advances in diagnostics and the understanding of the various conditions that affect the auditory system. Each auditory pathology can manifest distinct audible behaviors and needs, requiring individualized therapeutic approaches. Hence, the objective of this chapter is to explore the various therapeutic possibilities available, which include not only the use of hearing devices but also adaptive methodologies and therapeutic approaches aimed at auditory rehabilitation in different clinical scenarios specifically auditory neuropathy, Down syndrome, non-progressive chronic encephalopathies, and autism. Interventions can vary from the use of hearing aids suitable for the patient's auditory profile to rehabilitation programs that incorporate auditory stimulation techniques and social skills training, which are essential for the overall development of these children, as well as the inclusion of bilingual plans using sign language. The importance of an accurate diagnosis and the definition of an appropriate rehabilitation plan are fundamental to maximizing the effectiveness of these interventions. Additionally, approaches such as hearing rehabilitation techniques, listening training, and communication-centered interventions can complement the use of devices and provide a holistic approach to rehabilitation. It is essential to consider cultural and educational factors in the treatment process, as these aspects can influence the adaptation and success of each individual's auditory rehabilitation. This requires collaborative work among professionals from different areas, such as audiologists, speech therapists, occupational therapists, and educators, along with the family, to develop a therapeutic plan that meets specific needs.

Keywords: hearing impairment, auditory rehabilitation, hearing devices, family support, childhood

1. Introduction

The generalization of auditory rehabilitation is no longer acceptable today, especially considering the substantial advancements in diagnostics and the understanding of various conditions that affect the auditory system. Each auditory pathology can manifest distinct behaviors and rehabilitation needs, necessitating individualized therapeutic approaches.

The World Health Organization (WHO) [1] and the Gallaudet Institute [2] indicate that approximately 20%–40% of children with hearing impairments have some significant additional disability. Auditory rehabilitation should be considered part of a multidisciplinary process, recognizing that each child has unique characteristics and needs that influence their rehabilitation journey. The diagnosis of hearing loss and associated impairments may not always be evident and requires ongoing monitoring.

Identifying the type, degree, and configuration of hearing loss in children with other comorbidities is not an easy task and requires the principle of cross-checking, which consists of a battery of tests for pediatric auditory assessment, complementing behavioral tests and electrophysiological evaluations. To this end, it is essential to ensure that the middle ear is in good condition, as well as overall health, and to consider cognitive, socio-emotional, and other factors [3].

Consequently, in some cases, it is not always possible to commence auditory rehabilitation by the age of three months, as recommended by the Joint Committee on Infant Hearing [4], due to various factors contributing to the delay in diagnosing deafness.

Auditory rehabilitation, which includes the use of hearing aids (HA), cochlear implants (CI), bone-anchored hearing aids (BAHA), and timely intervention programs, is essential for children with hearing loss and other comorbidities, as these children may experience significant delays in language, speech, cognitive, and psychosocial development, among others.

In this context, the purpose of this chapter is to explore the various therapeutic possibilities available, which include not only the use of auditory devices but also adaptive methodologies and therapeutic approaches aimed at auditory rehabilitation, language, and communication across different clinical scenarios.

2. Adequate rehabilitation plans are fundamental to maximize the effectiveness of these interventions – overview

Therapeutic planning in the context of therapy for children with hearing loss and other comorbidities is configured as a collaborative process that emerges from an understanding of the child's history, possibilities, needs, and interests, along with those of their family [5, 6]. The development of the therapeutic plan involves a person-centered approach, the expertise of the professional, and the involvement of the family. At this stage, the collected information is carefully integrated and transformed into concrete strategies that will be applied in the family routine, aiming to promote a true exchange of experiences.

Regarding therapeutic strategies, the goal is to expand the child's linguistic-communicative repertoire and social relationships. To achieve this, a structured set of guidelines and dynamics is established to inform the sessions, creating a safe and accessible space that aims not only to meet specific demands but also to foster an environment conducive to mutual learning and development. In this context, there is an emphasis on respecting and valuing the uniqueness of each child and their family, thus recognizing the importance of individuality in the therapeutic process and strengthening the relationship of trust and collaboration.

Adapting techniques to align with the child's developmental level and therapeutic goals is essential for promoting an effective learning environment. This involves considering the child's cognitive, emotional, and physical capabilities, ensuring that the proposed activities are challenging, and emphasizing the importance of a purpose-driven learning journey with established goals.

By customizing approaches, therapists can facilitate skill-building in a playful and engaging manner, fostering both confidence and motivation. Moreover, this adaptation allows interventions to become more relevant and impactful, which contributes to more significant and sustainable progress in the child's development.

3. Therapeutic approaches

3.1 Auditory–oral therapy

Auditory–oral therapy is an approach aimed at enhancing hearing and verbal communication in individuals with hearing impairments. By focusing on therapeutic situations, this technique sets interaction and spoken language stimulation goals, adapting to the specific needs of each patient. Electronic devices such as HA, CI, and BAHA are essential tools in this process. They not only improve sound perception but also assist in language practice in various contexts [7–9]. The establishment of short-, medium-, and long-term goals provides a clear direction for treatment. Each goal can include various strategies, such as active listening activities, interactive games, and structured conversations that promote the development of spoken language. Additionally, the work is family-centered, which is crucial for creating a supportive and motivating environment [6].

3.2 Bilingualism

Bilingualism, understood as the ability to establish a meaningful relationship between spoken language and sign language, goes beyond the simple verbal/gestural articulation. Being bilingual implies not only fluency in two forms of communication but also active participation in both communities: that of hearing individuals and the deaf culture. This interaction deeply benefits the individual, providing a deeper understanding of the cultural nuances that permeate each group. The practice of bilingualism thus extends beyond the exchange of words – whether spoken or signed – and involves a commitment to respecting and valuing the cultural identities that each language represents. Therefore, bilingualism becomes a powerful means of promoting inclusion and mutual understanding among various ways of expressing and experiencing reality [10].

3.3 Augmentative and alternative communication

Augmentative and alternative communication (AAC) is a practice aimed at assisting individuals with difficulties in oral language to communicate more effectively. This approach encompasses both strategies and tools that help address the communication challenges faced by individuals with one or more impairments, including visual, auditory, sensory–motor, motivational, cognitive, linguistic, literacy skills, and current modes of communication. The tools of AAC vary widely, including materials ranging from graphics specifically developed for this purpose to resources such as photos and written texts. These graphic symbols can be organized through rudimentary and high-tech resources, from simple sheets of paper to devices like computers and tablets. The use of these tools is accompanied by clinical and pedagogical actions aiming to facilitate access and the creation of symbols that transform into means of communication [11].

A fundamental principle of AAC is the idea that communication is not limited to speech. It can be expressed through various modes, such as gestures, manual signs, finger spelling, facial expressions, tangible objects, communication boards, touch, writing, and pointing to symbols or images, as well as using electronic devices like HA, CI, and BAHA, or even speech-generating devices. This allows individuals to interact in varied ways, promoting more inclusive and effective communication [11, 12]

4. Intervention in various diagnoses of deafness and other comorbidities

4.1 Non-evolving chronic encephalopathy

Non-evolving chronic encephalopathy (NECE) is characterized as a stable sequela of dysfunctions in the central nervous system, occurring at various stages of development: prenatal, perinatal, and postnatal. The etiology of NECE is multifactorial, involving genetic or hereditary aspects during the prenatal period and various factors in the perinatal phase, such as circulatory-ischemic events, intracranial hemorrhages, gestational immaturity, and neonatal asphyxia or anoxia. In the postnatal context, the condition can be exacerbated by infections like viral or bacterial meningitis, as well as craniocephalic trauma, which significantly impacts the child's neurological development.

A study conducted by Levy and Rosenberg [13] evaluated the auditory function of 46 children diagnosed with NECE, regardless of the presence of auditory complaints. The results indicated that 52% of participants exhibited some degree of hearing loss, with the most common causes related to encephalopathies and hypoxic-ischemia, followed by infectious processes, kernicterus, and congenital malformations. This evidence underscores the importance of thorough auditory evaluations to avoid underestimating these children's linguistic capabilities. Other studies have highlighted the performance in the development of both oral and gestural language, as well as the use of technology. Most studies conclude that many children can access auditory stimuli, which provides them with various advantages; however, it does not guarantee the development of spoken language [14, 15].

The relationship between hearing and language development is complex and multifaceted, making language delays an intriguing phenomenon. Delays in acquiring linguistic skills can be attributed to various factors, including neurological impairments that affect cognitive abilities and auditory processing, as well as specific characteristics of hearing loss that can vary in type and degree. In many cases, it is challenging to determine whether the linguistic delay is a result of underlying neurological dysfunctions or a direct consequence of the nature of the hearing loss. Studies demonstrate that hearing plays a crucial role in language development, and a lack of appropriate auditory stimuli can significantly interfere with the acquisition of linguistic skills. Therefore, it is essential to conduct comprehensive and interdisciplinary assessments to discern the underlying causes of language delays, taking into account both auditory and neurological aspects [16, 17].

4.2 Down syndrome – trisomy of chromosome 21

Among chromosomal anomalies, Down syndrome (DS) is one of the most common, with an estimated occurrence of 1 in every 700 live births. This genetic alteration affects various aspects of development and has significant implications, including a likelihood of hearing impairment. Studies indicate that approximately 75% of children with trisomy 21 may experience hearing loss, although the incidence of congenital hearing loss is relatively rare. The main otological factors affecting this population include functional and anatomical anomalies of the eustachian tube, narrowing of the acoustic meatus, secretory otitis media, alterations in the ossicular chain, and malformations of the inner ear. These characteristics are associated with hearing impairment, whose incidence varies, with estimates ranging from 8% to 82% of cases [18].

Given the various factors that a child with DS may face, there are numerous complications that impact their development, including hearing loss, which can be either temporary or permanent. Temporary hearing losses, often related to ear infections or anatomical factors, may significantly interfere with incidental learning, which is crucial for the acquisition of skills and knowledge. Without proper monitoring and the implementation of strategies that promote a suitable learning environment, these auditory limitations can hinder the child's ability to communicate and interact. In the long run, this can lead to significant educational and social challenges, compromising incidental learning if there is no effective follow-up and strategies in place to improve learning conditions.

It is essential that a multidisciplinary team collaborates to promote better outcomes for children with DS. This team should focus on providing comprehensive auditory assessments, interventions, and educational strategies tailored to the child's individual needs, ensuring that they can thrive both academically and socially.

4.3 Autism spectrum disorder

The prevalence of autism in deaf children is a topic that deserves attention, as both conditions can interact in complex ways. Research suggests that while 1%–2% of deaf children and youth may have autism spectrum disorder (ASD), the lack of precise data regarding this specific population poses a challenge for accurate identification and diagnosis. It is crucial for health and education professionals to be aware of the particularities that may arise when autism symptoms are presented in children with hearing loss. These children may exhibit communication and social interaction difficulties that manifest differently due to the sensory barrier of deafness [19, 20].

Moreover, the high rates of comorbidities among autistic and deaf children indicate a need for a multidisciplinary approach to diagnosis and treatment. Providing adequate support for communication development, whether through sign language or alternative communication methods, can be vital in helping these children thrive [21, 22].

Planning for a child's communication development should take into account their receptive and expressive language levels, among other factors. In terms of receptive language, the child may recognize isolated words, understand short everyday phrases, follow simple one-step instructions with visual cues, and respond to basic questions. For expression, the child may communicate through gestures, such as pulling hands, using isolated words, sign language, or utilizing AAC devices. Additionally, evaluating the usage, timing, and comfort levels of auditory devices like HA or CI is important. It is essential to know sensory triggers that could cause discomfort, such as loud noises or uncomfortable environments.

To facilitate understanding and reduce anxiety, teamwork is crucial. Various studies highlight the benefits of CI for deaf children with autism, noting improvements in receptive language; however, this does not always guarantee progress in expressive language. Therefore, a tailored approach that considers the unique needs of children with both deafness and autism is essential for fostering their communication skills and overall development [23–26].

4.4 Auditory neuropathy

With a prevalence of 7%–10%, auditory neuropathy (AN) is a significant cause of sensorineural hearing loss [27]. Also known as AN spectrum disorder (ANSD), it occurs when there are disruptions in the neural synchronization of inner hair cells or the auditory neural pathways, while the function of outer hair cells remains normal. The characteristics of AN include fluctuation in hearing, sensitivity in tonal thresholds, reduced speech perception performance – especially in challenging auditory situations such as noisy environments – and decreased sound localization abilities [28].

The communication strategies adopted in the therapeutic process are influenced by the historical moment of identifying AN in childhood. Strategic choices are also determined by the topodiagnostic characteristics of the auditory alteration. Some auditory changes can impact the temporal aspects of speech and frequency discrimination, while sensorineural hearing loss affects the perception of frequency and/or intensity. Therefore, it is not feasible to predict the degree of difficulty in speech comprehension solely based on an audiological examination. In cases where neural alterations are significant, speech recognition abilities may be compromised, particularly in noisy environments.

The recommendation for HA appears to offer fewer benefits compared to CI. However, when the goal is to promote the development of speech and language, there is no guarantee that any device will be effective. Therefore, it is essential to conduct trials with HA and evaluate for cochlear implantation while emphasizing the need for rigorous follow-up. This comprehensive approach ensures that the unique needs of the child with AN are addressed effectively, facilitating the best possible outcomes in communication and language development [29, 30].

5. Challenges and benefits

Auditory rehabilitation in difficult cases must be deeply aligned with the rights of inclusion and equity, reflecting the principles of inclusive education promoted by UNESCO (2009). This process is vital for recognizing and addressing the diverse needs of each child, ensuring that their participation in social and educational environments is both effective and meaningful.

Thus, the aim is to promote accessible rehabilitation for all through the necessary adaptations, structures, and individual strategies that respect diversity.

Furthermore, the Convention on the Rights of Persons with Disabilities (CRPD) reinforces the importance of ensuring dignity, autonomy, non-discrimination, and equal opportunities. By ensuring that individuals with hearing impairments and other comorbidities have access to essential life skills and social development, we emphasize the need for inclusive support. Therefore, auditory rehabilitation in difficult cases is not just about improving hearing; it is a fundamental step to ensure that all children can learn, fully participate in daily life, and consequently have their voices heard in society.

6. Final considerations

Auditory rehabilitation in children with special needs must integrate all aspects discussed in this document, emphasizing the importance of a structured and collaborative plan.

First and foremost, it is essential that the objectives – short-term, medium-term, and long-term – are clear and tailored to the reality of each child. Auditory rehabilitation should have specific goals that allow for tracking progress and adjusting interventions when necessary.

Family involvement is a fundamental pillar in this process. It is crucial that family members understand and actively participate in the rehabilitation plan, as this strengthens emotional and practical support for the child. Furthermore, being a good listener to families and understanding their needs helps personalize the treatment according to individual requirements, thus establishing a bond of trust.

The role of a multidisciplinary team is vital. Collaboration among healthcare professionals, families, and schools ensures a holistic approach, enabling all areas related to the child's development to be considered. The integration of educational and medical interventions provides better adaptation and acceptance of auditory devices, when indicated, which should be selected and adjusted according to each child's specific hearing needs.

Willingness to change is an important characteristic in the rehabilitation process, as the child's needs may evolve over time. As such, regularly reviewing and adapting interventions will ensure that rehabilitation remains effective.

Finally, it is essential to identify each child's potential and celebrate their accomplishments, however small. The focus should not only be on difficulties but also on the skills that can be developed. By joining efforts to achieve comprehensive and mindful hearing rehabilitation, it is possible to provide a significant improvement in the quality of life for these children.

Beyond overcoming barriers, fostering an exchange of experiences among parents, children, therapists, and the multidisciplinary team is a project that seeks to challenge limitations and celebrate achievements.

Author details

Cilmara Cristina Alves da Costa Levy
Vice- President of the Brasilian Academy of Audiology (2025–2027), Brasilian Academy of Audiology, São Paulo, Brazil

*Address all correspondence to: Cilmara.levy@gmail.com

References

[1] OMS WHO. Deafness and Hearing Loss. Who.int. Available online: https://www.who.int/news-room/fact-sheets/detail/deafness-and-hearing-loss [Accessed: 2025-September-06]

[2] Gallaudet Research Institute. (2011). Regional and national summary report of data from the 2009–2010 annual survey of deaf and hard of hearing children and youth.

[3] Hall III JW. Crosscheck principle in pediatric audiology today: A 40-year perspective. Journal of Audiology and Otology. 2016;**20**(2):59–67. DOI: 10.7874/jao.2016.20.2.59

[4] Joint Committee on Infant Hearing 2019. The Journal of Early Hearing Detection and Intervention. 2019; **4**(2):1–44

[5] Rhoades EA. Serving families with diverse cultures. In: Roades EA, Ducan J, editors. Auditory-Verbal Pracitice: Family- Centered Early Interventio 2 nd. Springfild IL: Charles C Thomas; 2017. p. 78–102

[6] Melo ME, and CCAC L. Abordagem Centrada na Família de Serviços fonoaudiológicos para bebês e crianças pequenas surdas em Levy CCAC. In Manual de Audiologia Pediatrico. Vol. 1. 2 edn. São Paulo: Manole; 2022. p. 11

[7] Bevilacqua MC, Formigoni GMP. Audiologia Educacional: Uma Opção Terapêutica Para Crianças Deficientes Auditiva. 1 ed. Curitiba: Pro-Fono; 1997. p. 86p

[8] Estabrooks W, M-lk MHM. Auditory-verbal Therapy: Science, Research, and Practice. San Diego: Plural; 2020

[9] Levy CCAC, Formigon GMP, Brazorotto JS. Ntervenção fonoaudiológica na reabilitação auditiva infantil. Eliane S. Vol. 1, et al. Tratado de Audiologia. Available From: VitalSource Bookshelf. 3rd. São Paulo Editora Manole; 2022. p. 612–631

[10] Bergrow Ddi V, Brito LT. Aquisição de linguagem e o contexto linguistico da criança surda in Cecilia Moura (Editor). Desirée De Vit Begrow Libras e surdos. Finalista Jabuti Acadêmico políticas: linguagem e inclusão; 2025

[11] Augmentative and Alternative Communication (AAC) Available from: https://www.asha.org/practice-portal/professional-issues/augmentative-and-alternative-communication/ [Accessed: 2025-September-14]

[12] Available from: https://www.isaacbrasil.org.br/comunicaccedilatildeo-aumentativa-e-alternativa.html [Accessed: 2025-September-14]

[13] Levy CCAC, Rosemberg S. Crianças com encefalopatia crônica não evolutiva: Avaliação audiológica e próteses auditivas. Pró-Fono Revista de Atualização Científica. 2009;**21** (3):237–242. DOI: 10.1590/S0104-56872009000300010

[14] Cupples L, Ching TYC, Button L, Leigh G, Marnane V, Whitfield J, Gunnourie M, Martin L. Language and speech outcomes of children with hearing loss and additional disabilities: Identifying the variables that influence performance at five years of age. International Journal of Audiology.

2018;**57**(sup2):S93–S104. DOI: 10.1080/14992027.2016.1228127

[15] Lanphere A, Terlektsi E. Necessidades de comunicação de uma criança surda com paralisia cerebral e como apoiá-las: Um estudo de caso. Surdez E Educação Internacional. 2022;**25**(2):101–120. DOI: 10.1080/14643154.2022.2133386

[16] Findlen U, Richard C. Hearing and speech interactions in children with cerebral palsy, in the first 2 years: Focus on cerebral palsy. Pediatric Research. 2024. DOI: 10.1038/s41390-024-03403-0

[17] Levy CCAC, Sousa Neto OM. Intervenções nas alterações auditivas: Encefalopatia crônica não evolutiva e deficiência auditiva. In Boechat EM, Menezes PL, Couto CM, Fizzo ACF, Scharlach RC, Anastasio ART. Tratado de Audiologia. 2. ed. Rio de Janeiro: Guanabara Koogan; 2015. p. 489–494

[18] Documento científico. Departamento científico de otorrinolaringologia (gestão 2022-2024). Sociedade Brasileira de Pediatria N. 2024;**160**:27. https://www.sbp.com.br/fileadmin/user_upload/sbp/2024/agosto/14/24493e-DocCient_-_Sindrome_Down_e_a_OtorrinoPediatrica.pdf?

[19] American Psychiatry Association (APA). Manual Diagnóstico E Estatístico de Transtornos mentais-DSM-V. Porto Alegre: Artmed; 2014

[20] Whitehouse A, Evans K, Eapen V, Prof A, Wray J A national guideline for the assessment and diagnosis of autism spectrum disorders in Australia 2018. Available from: https://www.autismcrc.com.au [Accessed: 2025-December]

[21] Brasil. Ministério da saúde. secretaria de atenção à saúde. departamento de atenção especializada e temática. linha de cuidado para a atenção às pessoas com transtorno do espectro do autismo e suas famílias na rede de atenção psicossocial do sistema único de saúde [Internet]. 2015. undefined–156. Available from: https://www.saude.gov.br [Accessed: 2025-December]

[22] Centers for Disease Control and Prevention. Information from your family doctor: Autism spectrum disorder. What is autism spectrum disorder? Can vaccines cause ASD? [Internet]. 2016. Available from: https://www.cdc.gov/autism/faq/index.html

[23] Eshraghi AA, Nazarian R, Telischi FF, Martinez D, Hodges A, Velandia S, Cejas-Cruz I, Balkany TJ, Lo K, Lang D. cochlear implantation in children with autism spectrum disorder. Otology and Neurotology. 2015;**36**(8):e121–8. DOI: 10.1097/MAO.0000000000000757

[24] Tavares FS. Implante coclear em pacientes com Transtorno do Espectro Autista : revisão sistemática Dissertação (mestrado). Universidade de Brasília, Faculdade de Ciências da Saúde, Programa de Pós-Graduação em Ciências da Saúde; 2021. https://repositorio.unb.br/handle/10482/43145?locale=en

[25] Fidencio VLD, Silva JM, Souza TM, Vicente LC, Ribeiro CC Luders D. Avalição e resultado de crianças usuarias de implante coclear com transtorno do espectro autista? Revisao integrativa da literatura. Revista CEFAC. 2023;**25**(5):e5223. DOI: 10.1590/1982-0216/20232555223s

[26] Lachowska M, Pastuszka A, Lukaszewicz-Moszynska Z,

Mikolajewska L, Niemczyk K. Cochlear implantation in autistic children with profound sensorineural hearing loss. Brazilian Journal of Otorhinolaryngology. 2018;**84**(1):15–19

[27] Ehrmann-Müller D, Cebulla M, Rak K, Scheich M, Back D, Hagen R, Shehata-Dieler W. Evaluation and therapy outcome in children with auditory neuropathy spectrum disorder (ANSD). International Journal of Pediatric Otorhinolaryngology. 2019;**127**:109681. DOI: 10.1016/j.ijporl.2019.109681

[28] Starr A. Rance G. Chapter 28 Auditory neuropathy. Handbook of Clinical Neurology. 2015;**129**:495–508. DOI: 10.1016/B978-0-444-62630-1.00028-7

[29] Morlet T, O'Reilly R, Pritchett C, Venskytis E, Parkes W. A 15-year review of 260 children with auditory neuropathy spectrum disorder: II. Management and Outcomes. Ear Hear. 2023;**44**(5):979–989. DOI: 10.1097/AUD.0000000000001366

[30] Mesallam TA, Yousef M, Almasaad A. Auditory and language skills development after cochlear implantation in children with multiple disabilities. European Archives of Oto-Rhino-Laryngology. 2019;**276**(1):49–55. DOI: 10.1007/s00405-018-5184-0